☞ **W9-DFN-074**

MNEMONICS AND TACTICS
IN SURGERY AND MEDICINE

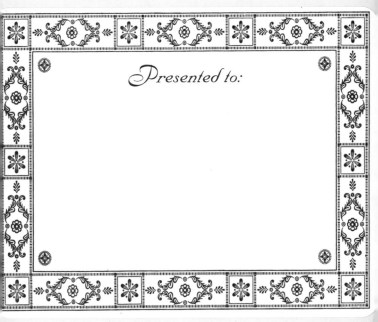

Presented to:

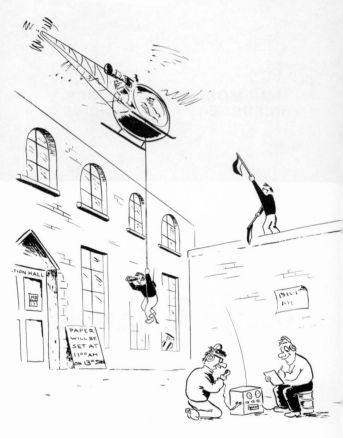

TACTICS EARN M.D.

Mnemonics and Tactics in Surgery and Medicine

John J. Shipman
M.B., L.R.C.P., M.S.(Lond.), F.R.C.S.(Eng.)

Senior Consultant Surgeon
The Lister Hospital, Stevenage, and Associated Hospitals

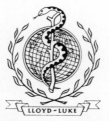

LLOYD-LUKE (MEDICAL BOOKS) LTD
49 NEWMAN STREET
LONDON
1978

PRINTED AND BOUND IN ENGLAND BY
HAZELL WATSON AND VINEY LTD
AYLESBURY, BUCKS

ISBN 0 85324 135 X

DEDICATED TO ALL LONG-SUFFERING STUDENTS

*   *   *

We'll refuse to remember mnemonics,
We'll fail and be happy as chronics.

Richard Leech
World Medicine
9th March, 1977

PREFACE

The aspiring medical student is confronted with a rapidly accumulating mass of information and is expected to memorize a considerable amount of it. The easiest way to do so, if the subject allows, is to understand it and to work out a logical sequence. Here physiology and pathology are invaluable. Anatomy apart from other considerations may provide a classification. Seeing and examining patients with various diseases, viewing slides, X-rays and clinical pictures is part of the training; practical work cannot be superseded.

However, lists must be learnt including the order of frequency. To help memorize the lists, classifications must be learnt. The letters of the phrase "Tactics earn M.D." provide a large number of headings relating to possible causes, and it, or something similar, must be learnt.

The treatment of any disease depends on a number of variables and in order to jog the memory "Cages" or the "Cs" is introduced — the letters referring to the possible variables. Aetiology, too, contains innumerable factors and "I'm chaste" may help. In the presentation of a disease, the use of words beginning with an "S" will open up extensive variations. It is often important to know how many facts need to be learnt and the "Fives" are illustrated. In the diagnosis of a condition "Bed-side tests" are emphasized.

Symptoms and signs of disease may be remembered if the various systems are considered; an attempt has been made to identify those areas usually omitted.

Are there other ways of aiding memory? I was impressed by the use of the mnemonic "Parkinson's" for Parkinson's disease told to me by Mr Alan Mullins, a Surgeon from Australia and at one time my Registrar, and since that time I have busied myself making my own and stimulating the Royal Free students to do likewise. It is a most amusing mental exercise, aids memory, and is warmly recommended.

The book contains many examples. Some are like *The Times* crossword; others, like "Fred can't stop . . .", do not require difficult memory feats. One of the problems is to form a memory aid in the order of frequency and this is more difficult. Practical work in hospital should provide information regarding the first three probables and some important features in the mnemonics are marked with an asterisk.

As a surgeon, I have with considerable trepidation entered the world of medicine. Here the information is so complex that the opportunity for creating mnemonics is boundless.

Students create for themselves summaries, diagrams and rhymes during their hospital training, and it is hoped that the effective ones will be sent in as they are created. Even if some efforts are made to form them and only a few are remembered, particularly the classifications, the author feels that despite the unorthodox methods described the work done will have been justified.

I would like to express my appreciation for the help, encouragement and advice given to me by present and former members of the staff of the Lister Hospital, including P. J. Mills, F.R.C.P., Roger Armour, Ch.M., F.R.C.S., J. R. B. Williams, M.D., F.R.C.Path., W. E. Essigman, M.R.C.P., M. G. Hoffman, M.R.C.O.G., F.R.C.S.(Eng. & Edin.), T. H. To, M.B., B.S., B. M. Newman, M.D., F.R.C.S., A. E. Mullins, M.B.(Aust.), F.R.C.S., Mrs M. P. Stainton, Ph.C., M.P.S. and J. Atwood, S.R.N. I would particularly like to thank Paul Siklos, M.R.C.P. and Alison Early, M.R.C.P. for reading through the text and offering helpful suggestions.

Thanks are also due to the enthusiastic students of the Royal Free Hospital who have attended the Lister Hospital for two weeks as part of their surgical training and who have helped in the creation of some of the mnemonics, my secretaries, Mrs Vera Holloway and Mrs H. Wendy Miller, and, for the cartoons so skilfully drawn, Mr Michael Flemming.

CONTENTS

LIST OF ABBREVIATIONS

ACTH	Adrenocorticotrophic hormone
ADH	Anti-diuretic hormone
a-v	Arteriovenous
CCF	Congestive cardiac failure
CIX	Cystine indigo xanthine
CNS	Central nervous system
CSF	Cerebrospinal fluid
CVA	Cerebrovascular accident
DLE	Disseminated lupus erythematosus
DS	Disseminated sclerosis
DVT	Deep venous thrombosis
ECG	Electrocardiogram
ESR	Erythrocyte sedimentation rate
FB	Foreign body
GPI	General paralysis of the insane
Hb	Haemoglobin
IgA	Immunoglobulin A
IgD	Immunoglobulin D
IgE	Immunoglobulin E
IgG	Immunoglobulin G
IgM	Immunoglobulin M
IVC	Inferior vena cava
LATS	Long-acting thyroid stimulator
LDH	Lactate dehydrogenase
LE	Lupus erythematosus
LV	Left ventricle
MI	Mitral incompetence
MSH	Melanocyte-stimulating hormone
MSU	Midstream specimen of urine
Po_2	Partial pressure of oxygen
RBC	Red blood cell
SBE	Subacute bacterial endocarditis
SLE	Systemic lupus erythematosus
TSH	Thyroid-stimulating hormone
VMA	Vanillylmandelic acid
WBC	White blood-cell count

*Some important features in the mnemonics are marked with an asterisk.

CHAPTER 1

GENERAL SUBJECTS

Causes

There are a variety of ways that can be used to list causes; the following phrase is recommended and should be learnt thoroughly:

"TACTICS EARN M.D., Gertrude."

Tumours.
> Innocent; Single and multiple. Malignant; Primary; carcinoma (melanoma), sarcoma, teratoma, hormone-producing or inactive. Secondary; Hormone-producing or inactive.

Accidents.
> Blunt; Penetrating injuries with or without the presence of a foreign body. Note: FB should remind you of gall-stone, swallowed bone, etc.
> Rays; too hot, too cold (frostbite), too much irradiation.
> Doctors, surgeons, and their complications.

Congenital.

Topical and Tropical. Topical refers to lesions particular to the part,
> e.g. hydrocele in scrotum, hiatus hernia as a cause of dysphagia.

Inflammations. Include infections and allergies. Note: start small and increase the size of the pathogen. Viruses, Rickettsiae, bacteria, fungi, protozoa, parasites. Remember tuberculosis may affect all tissues. Think of Crohn's or ulcerative colitis. These diseases are inflammations, not infections.

Collagen Disease.

Syphilis.

Endocrine. From above downwards: pituitary, thyroid and parathyroid, thymus, pancreas and adrenals, gonads and possibly kidneys and placenta.

Anaemias. Arteries, veins, lymphatics and heart.

Reticuloses. Connect with "Tumours" and include leukaemias.

Nervous. Psychological and true nervous diseases.

Metabolic. Myopathies, mechanical causes, e.g. intussusceptions, adhesions.

Diet. Drugs, poisons and degeneration (e.g., osteoarthritis).

Gertrude. Gynaecological causes.

Describe the Causes of Dysphagia

If this subject is for discussion, the following routine may be considered:

(1) First write down in note form all the information that can be memorized;

(2) Draw a rough sketch of the anatomy;

(3) Think of the tube variables — "in the wall, in the lumen and outside".

Then go through "Tactics" etc. We will start with "Tactics".

Tumours. Any tumour, innocent or malignant, single or multiple, arising in or implicating the oropharynx, hypopharynx, or oesophagus, may cause dysphagia. Leiomyoma is the commonest innocent tumour of the oesophagus.

Accidents. Any blunt or penetrating injury from the mouth downwards causing swelling, haematoma, ulceration, then possibly stricture, may produce dysphagia. A swallowed, impacted foreign body is a potent cause. Burns due to accidentally or deliberately swallowed corrosives, burns of the mouth and tongue, irradiation damage coincident with irradiation, say, of a carcinoma of the thyroid. Any endoscopy or operation on the pharynx, or oesophagoscopy followed by inflammation, ulceration, leakage, stricture, will result in this symptom.

Congenital. Stenosis may occur or follow repair of fistulae. Abnormally placed vessels may produce pressure effects. Diaphragmatic hernia may be a cause.

Tropical and Topical. Chagas' disease (trypanosomiasis). Topical is, of course, hiatus hernia with regurgitant oesophagitis, ulceration, spasm and stricture. Achalasia of the oesophagus.

Infection. Any virus, fungus, bacterium, causing inflammation etc. of the pharynx or oesophagus.
Collagen Diseases. Scleroderma.
Syphilis may produce lesions in the oropharynx and of course aneurysms.

Endocrine. Thyroid enlargements in the tongue, neck or mediastinum, parathyroid enlargements. Similarly other intrathoracic neoplasms may produce dysphagia if the oesophagus becomes implicated.
Anaemias. Arteries and veins, etc. Plummer-Vinson (Paterson-Kelly) syndrome is a cause. Dilated veins. Aneurysms from other causes.
Reticuloses. Gland enlargements or implication of pharynx or oesophagus may result in dysphagia.
Nervous lesions. Hysteria, bulbar lesions, diphtheria, tetanus, DS.

Metabolic. Uraemia.
Myopathies. Myasthenia gravis.
Mechanical. Pharyngeal pouch.
Drugs. Retropleural fibrosis may occur.

Many causes may be gleaned by such a consideration. It is emphasized that the object of this book is to facilitate the recall of a series of disjointed facts.

Diagnosis of "X"

How do you diagnose a condition?

Unfortunately, during the examination the most important investigations are left unstated, and it is to emphasize their omission that the following statement is made, i.e. "Bedside Tests".

The diagnosis depends on:

(1) The history.
(2) Clinical examination.
(3) Bedside tests. *These include temperature, pulse, respiration, blood pressure, urine,* examination of stools, vomitus and sputum*.
(4) Other investigations: radiology, blood tests, etc.

* Asterisks mark essential points or those most easily forgotten.

Examination Questions in Pathology

To answer a general question in pathology, the following phrase may be useful:

"Ian Aird said good pathologists make mighty surgeons pleased."

Incidence.
Age.
Sex.
Geographical factors.
Predisposing factors.
Macroscopy.
Microscopy.
Spread.
Prognosis.

Inventor unknown.

THE TREATMENT. "CAGES"

Treatment of all Conditions

How do you treat a given condition?
The treatment depends on the variables in the word:

"CAGES"

Complications — the presence or absence thereof.
Age.
General conditions, e.g. recent coronary thrombosis precludes surgery.
Etiology (American spelling).
Site, symptoms and stage.

Note: Etiology should be emphasized first.

Example: How do you treat a gastric ulcer?
It depends on: the etiology (it may be malignant); the age and general condition of the patient; the presence or absence of complications such as perforation, bleeding or gastric stenosis; the severity of symptoms etc.

To give examples, simple ones first:

If a patient presents with a chronic gastric ulcer, is otherwise fit, and does not respond to medical treatment, surgery such as a Billroth I partial gastrectomy is recommended.

If a patient presents with a perforated gastric ulcer, a laparotomy is performed after resuscitation and the perforation is closed.

If the defect is too large and the patient is fit enough, a partial gastrectomy is performed.

If a patient presents with an hour-glass stomach, a partial gastrectomy is undertaken after the patient's general condition has been improved, etc.

Treatment of Any Condition

An alternative to answering a question on treatment is to use the words below that begin with the letter "C"; note this introduces the word *Cause* first, which is correct. How do you treat a condition? It depends on:

FIVE Cs

Cause.*
Course.
Complications.
Condition of patient.
Complaints.

Aetiology

CAUSES

Primary cause.
Precipitating factors.
Predisposing factors.
Associated conditions.

Variables are seen in

"I'M CHASTE"

Incidence.
Mendelian factors.

Congenital defects.
Habitat, e.g. lice.
Age.
Sex.
Topo- or geographical.
Economic, ethnological.

Classification of Investigations

A.B.C.D.E.F.

Anatomy, morbid. Biopsy and histology, cytology.
Bacteriology. Immunology; animal inoculation; micro-
    biology; sensitivity to antiobiotics.
Chemistry. Constituents; uptakes; excretion.
Diagnostic radiology. X-rays; isotopes; scanning.
Endoscopy and exploration.
Full blood and marrow counts.

Characteristics of Pain

It is essential to learn the variations of pain.

"NEVER STOPS"

Nature.
Easing and precipitating factors.
Vomiting.
External manifestations — redness, hyperaesthesia.
Radiation.

Site and severity.
Time, duration.
Onset.
Prodromal factors, posture.
Shock, sequelae, sweating.

Classification of Systems

To remember various symptoms of disease, use of the alphabet may help to cover the systems:

A to P

Alimentary. Anorexia, hiccups, distention, bowel irregularities, bleeding etc.

Blood. Anaemias, weakness, breathlessness, pallor. (Electrolytic changes, calcium, uric acid, sodium etc. and their features.)

Chest. Cardiac and pericardium.

Dermatological. Erythema nodosum, pigmentation etc.

Ear, nose and throat. Tongue, halitosis, buccal ulcers, dysphagia, sore throat etc.

Facies. e.g. Hippocratic.

Glands.

Hypertension manifestations. Headache etc.

Immunity effects.

Joints and bones.

Kidney and bladder.

Liver and legs, e.g. oedema.

Muscles.

Nervous system, central.

Ophthalmic.

Peripheral nerves.

Systemic effects.

An alternative aid is to consider head and neck. Head will remind you of facies, eye, ear, nose and throat, tongue, mouth ulcers, skin, bones and muscles; neck will remind you of glands, thyroid or parathyroid effects.

Examining Casualty

All patients are examined fully;* however, the following may jog the memory:

SEVEN Bs

Brain.
Beauty* (e.g. depressed zygoma*).
Bleeding.
Breathing.
Bowel.
Bladder.*
Bones.

Emergency Admissions

This aid may help the check-up:

"CLOTS"

Complications may be present. Look for nerve and
    arterial damage.
Losses. Assess the amount of blood or vomitus.
Obstructions. Check pharynx for obstructed airway*
    and bladder for retention.
Time.* Record the time that has elapsed since the
    injury.
Systemic effects. Check pulse, blood pressure, etc.

Fluids in the Various Compartments

Write down the numbers 1 2 3 4 5. Place a 0 below the 3. Then:

   0

   12 litres is the amount of interstitial fluid;

    3 litres is the plasma volume;

   30 litres in the cells;

   45 litres is the total.

Causes of Severe Loss of Weight
"WAISTED"

Whipple's disease, intestinal lipodystrophy (very rare), other causes of steatorrhoea.

Anorexia nervosa and depression.

Inflammations: tuberculosis, Crohn's, ulcerative colitis, subacute bacterial endocarditis.

Surgical: gut resections, stomach and bowel internal fistulae.

Tumours.

Endocrine: thyrotoxicosis, Addison's disease, Conn's syndrome, pituitary (Sheehan's).

Diabetes.

Effects of Nerve Injury
"SMART"

Sensory.

Motor.

Autonomic.

Reflex.

Trophic.

Causes of Glandular Enlargement

"STARS SIT"

Secondary carcinoma.
Tuberculosis.
Amyloid.
Reticuloses: Hodgkin's, etc.
Still's disease.

Sarcoidosis and syphilis.
Infective mononucleosis.*
Toxoplasmosis.

Postoperative Complications (1)

"JOHN SHIPMAN"

Jaundice, serum hepatitis, anaesthetic agents, mismatched blood transfusions.

Obstruction of bladder* or bowel, may be followed by wound dehiscence.

Haemorrhage and heart attack.

Neurological: brachial plexus, lithotomy injuries, senile dementia.

Shock and sepsis. Skin lesions, include bed-sores.

Hiccup, possibly uraemia.

Ileus, dilatation of stomach.

Pulmonary lesions: collapse of lung, embolus, abscess, pneumonia, foreign body swallowed, asthma attack.

Metabolic upsets: coma due to myxoedema, low potassium, sodium, dehydration.

Anuria.

Nausea and vomiting.

Not invented by Author.

Mnemonics and Tactics

Postoperative Complications (2)

"RATIONALISES SPACE"

Rotations: volvulus.
Acute gastric dilatation.
Thrombosis: occurring in the lower extremity, pelvis or
    mesenteric veins.
Infarcts.
Obstructions of bowel. Ileus.
Neurological, e.g. precipitates senile dementia.
Adhesions.
Leaks: fistulae with or without skin excoriation.
Infection of wound, bladder, parotids.
Stoppage of urine.
Evisceration of abdominal contents.
Subphrenic abscess.

Swallowed foreign body, e.g. dentures.
Pneumonia.
Air embolism.
Collapse of lung due to mucous plug.
Emboli.

Postoperative Complications (3)

"CHEST PROFESSOR"

Collapse of lung.
Heart attack.
Embolus. Venous thrombosis.
Swallowed FB or vomit.
Tension pneumothorax.

Perforation.
Rupture of wound.
Obstruction of bowel.
Fistula.
Electrolyte problems.
Stricture.
Sepsis.
Ophthalmic injury.
Retention of urine.

Features of a Lump

TEN Ss

Size.
Shape.
Surface, include temperature.
Site: including depth.
Symptoms: soreness, itching.
Softness: fluctuation.
Squeezability e.g. haemangiomata.
Spread, e.g. melanoma satellites, local lymph glands.
Stethoscopy.
Sensations: thrill (a-v fistula).

Clinical Presentation of Malignant Tumour

It depends on Ss

Take, for example, carcinoma of the stomach. It depends on:

Site, e.g. near oesophagus or pylorus.
Stage at which it presents.
Size, may produce a mass.
Secondaries, present or absent.
Systemic and non-metastatic effects, e.g. loss of weight, secondary anaemia, hormone effects.
Source: may have followed polyposis of stomach or peptic ulcer. (Two per cent become malignant.)
Spread, may have ulcerated into colon.
Side-effects, that is, complications, e.g. bleeding, perforation.
Sequelae, e.g. strictures.

Or:

Effects of Primary.
Effects of secondaries.
Non-metastatic effects. Hormonal effects: thrombophlebitis.
General effects, e.g. loss of weight etc.

Manifestations of Internal Malignancy

"BAD SITE"

Bullous eruptions.
Acanthosis nigricans.
Dermatomyositis.

Skin flushing with carcinoids.
Ichthyosis.
Tylosis: hyperkeratosis of palms and soles.
Erythema gyratum.

Features of Shock

"SHOCKED"

Skin pale, hands cold and sweaty, or hot* and dry
   with endotoxic shock.
Hypotension.
Oedema of lung.
Circulatory collapse.
Kidney failure.
Ecchymoses and petechiae.
Disseminated intravascular clotting.

Varieties of Shock

"HAVE A DRIP, PAT"

Haemorrhagic.
Anaphylactoid.
Vasovagal: neurogenic.
Endocrine: Friderichsen-Waterhouse   syndrome
   (adrenal apoplexy), Addison's, diabetes.

Acute pump failure or tamponade.

Dehydration and fluid losses, vomiting, diarrhoea.
Retropleural or peritoneal irritation.
Infection: peritonitis, pancreatitis, endotoxic.
Poisons, overdose.

Plasma loss: insect or snake bites, compression
   injuries.
Arterial obstructions.
Trauma, burns.

Features of Haemorrhage

"TRAPS"

Thirst.
Restlessness.*
Air hunger.
Pulse rising, pressure falling, pallor increasing.
Sweating.

Features of Potassium

"POTASSIUM"

Protein breakdown of 1 gram of nitrogen releases 3 mEq of potassium. Plasma K below 3 is significant depletion.

Organic mercurials may result in renal loss.

Two or more grams (60 to 80 mmol) are required daily.

Aldosterone retains sodium and water; potassium is lost.

Smooth, striated and cardiac muscle are affected, and possible ileus, hypotonicity and arrhythmias respectively may result with hypokalaemia.

Secondary renal tubular damage follows loss of potassium; polyuria results.

Intracellular distribution (98 per cent).

Urine is main excretory pathway. Distal tubules excrete it.

Mucus has high K content; losses therefore are significant.

Causes of Elevated Potassium

"DRAT IT"

Drugs.
Renal causes, diminished excretion.
Addisonian crisis, deficient aldosterone.
Transfusion: K content of stored blood plasma is higher.

Injury: cells destroyed release K.
Treatment may be excessive. Great care is required.

Causes of Potassium Leaving Cells

"ASSES"

Acidosis, H ions move in.
Starvation, catabolism of cells.
Stress, catabolism of cells (postoperative).
Exercise, catabolism of cells.
Sodium chloride lost; K replaces it and is then excreted.

Causes of Hypokalaemia

"MADRAS"

Metabolic: cirrhosis, diabetic ketosis, prolonged acidosis.

Alimentary: reduced intake, gastric lavage, pyloric stenosis, bowel resections, colostomies, ileostomies, faecal fistulae, diarrhoea, purgation, rectal tumours, papillomas secreting mucus which contains potassium.

Drugs: insulin, diuretics, ACTH and corticosteroid therapy. Treatment of megaloblastic anaemia.

Renal: tubular acidosis, tubular necrosis and damage, Fanconi's syndrome.

Adrenal gland: hyperaldosteronism, Cushing's syndrome.

Skin: burns.

Note: Mucus has high potassium content.*

Elevated Uric Acid

"DANGER"

Drugs: chlorothiazide and derivatives.
Anaemia: polycythaemia and haemolytic anaemia.
Neoplasm: myeloid leukaemia.
Gout and pseudogout.
Endocrine causes: parathyroid tumour, myxoedema.
Renal damage: diminished glomerular filtration.

Causes of Elevated Alkaline Phosphatase

"NEOPLASM"

Neoplasia: primary.
Endocrine: hyperparathyroidism.
Osteomalacia and rickets.
Paget's disease of bone.
Liver: biliary obstructive disease.
Acute viral infections, e.g. infective mononucleosis.
Secondaries.
Metabolism of bone; any change therein.

Causes of Elevated Aldosterone

"CRASH"

Congestive heart failure.
Renal: nephrosis.
Adrenal: Conn's syndrome.
Shock.
Hypertension, malignant.

CHAPTER 2

STOMACH AND DUODENUM

Differential Diagnosis of
Upper-Abdominal Pain

For severe upper-abdominal pain:

"PERFORATED ABDOMEN"

Perforation of peptic or malignant ulcer, or inflammatory lesion of oesophagus, stomach, Meckel's diverticulum, small or large bowel, gall bladder, typhoid ulcer or aneurysm etc.

Acute pancreatitis.
Biliary colic.
Diaphragmatic pleurisy. Diabetes.
Obstructions.
Myocardial infarction.
Exacerbation of duodenal ulcer, enteritis.
Neurological causes: shingles, spinal tumour etc.

Add for some of the other severe abdominal pains:

"DEAREST"

Dissecting aneurysm.
Embolus, mesenteric.
Acute appendicitis.
Renal and ureteric colic.
Endocrine: parathyroid tumour, diabetes.
Strangulations, volvulus.
Tropical: amoebiasis, typhoid, sickle-cell anaemia.

Possible Causes of Peptic Ulcer

"CUT STOMACH OUT"

Crohn's disease.
Ulcerative colitis.
Tumours, parathyroid, Zollinger-Ellison, apudomas of other organs.

Smoking.
Toxaemia.
"O" Blood Group.
Megaloblastic anaemia (hypoplasia of mucosa).
Alcohol, aspirin and other drugs.
Curling's ulcer, cortisone and stress.
Hyperchlorhydria.

Obstruction or regurgitation at the pylorus (Capper).
Uraemia.
Types of work and personality.

Classification of Peptic Ulcers

"SONS"

Sites (five): oesophagus, stomach, duodenum, jejunum (anastomotic), Meckel's.
Onset: acute, subacute, chronic.
Number: single, multiple ulcers or erosions.
Shape: circular, oval, linear (Mallory-Weiss).

Perforated Peptic Ulcer

Depends on Ps

A puking patient, perspiring with punishingly severe pain, with pulse rising, pressure falling, peristalsis losing, pain descending with pressure, guarding all over abdomen, lying perfectly still with peritonitis.

Remember: The stillness* of peritonitis.
                The restlessness of haemorrhage.
                The writhings of colic.

Causes of Haematemesis (1)

There are a variety of ways to facilitate recall. Grouping into "Fives" is of use in the oral examination.

Five Groups of Condition Causing Haematemesis

1. *Ulcers*. Single or multiple; acute, subacute or chronic; simple or peptic from mouth to Meckel's area. Responsible for 85 per cent of haematemesis.

   Note that there are five sites of peptic ulceration, and they are, from above downwards:

   Oesophagus
   Stomach
   Duodenum
   Jejunum
   Adjacent to Meckel's diverticulum
2. *Tumours*. See the variables under "Tactics".
3. *Portal hypertension*. "In out, in out." Obstruction inside the liver or outside; inside the portal or hepatic veins or outside.
4. *Blood diseases*. Haemophilia, leukaemia, scurvy, etc.
5. *Medical diseases and their treatments*. Acute fevers, auto-immune diseases. Drugs*: aspirins, anticoagulants, cortisone, Indocid and other drugs for the treatment of rheumatism etc.

An alternative technique is to run through "Tactics" or the word "Doubts" (see below) and for the rare causes of haematemesis the word "Poem".

Causes of Haematemesis (2)

"DOUBTS"

Drugs.
Oesophageal lesion, e.g. portal hypertension, dia-
phragmatic hernia with ulceration.
Ulcers or uraemia.
Blood diseases.
Tumours.
Swallowed blood.

Rare Causes of Haematemesis

"POEM"

Pseudoxanthoma elasticum.
Osler-Weber-Rendu syndrome.
Ehlers-Danlos syndrome.
Mallory-Weiss tears around oesophagus.

Complications of Gastrectomy

(1) Classify:
    (a) Early, intermediate or late.

    (b) Local and general complications, and those specific to the part.

(2) Or classify under Ds:

EIGHT Ds

Diarrhoea.
Dumping.
Dizziness.
Deficiencies – vitamins and iron.
Dysphagia.
Distension after meals.
Dilatation of remnant due to stenosis.
Debility.

Complications of Partial Gastrectomy

"STOMACH AFTER OPS"

Steatorrhoea.
Thinning (loss of weight).
Obstructions, adhesions, intussusceptions, torsions.
Malabsorption: deficiencies of vitamins B_{12} and C
   and iron.
Anaemias: micro- or macrocytic.
Calcium loss: osteoporosis.
Haemorrhages, hypoglycaemia.

Anastomotic ulcer.
Fistula into colon and/or small bowel.
Tuberculous chest infections are more liable to occur.
Emesis: bilious vomiting.
Rapid emptying with diarrhoea.

Over-full symptoms (distension) with normal meals.
Perforation of anastomotic ulcer or duodenal stump.
Sweating, stagnation, dumping.

Factors Possibly Predisposing to Carcinoma of Stomach

"STOMACH"

Spirits, smoking?

Topographical: Japan.

Other members of the family.

Megaloblastic anaemia, atrophic mucosa and achlorhydria.

"A" blood group.

Chronic gastric ulcer (2 per cent go malignant).

Hypertrophic gastritis.

Also polyposis of stomach.

Differential Diagnosis of the Three 'A's:

ANOREXIA, ASTHENIA and ANAEMIA

The symptoms of anorexia, asthenia, and anaemia occur early in particular diseases which are roughly situated in a circle around the abdomen.

Carcinoma of the stomach.

Carcinoma of pancreas.   Carcinoma of left colon,
                                                    splenic flexure.

Carcinoma of right colon.

Bladder, urinary tract.

Uraemia.

CHAPTER 3

SPLEEN

Functions of the Spleen

"RETRIAL"

Reticulo-endothelial function. It removes particulate matter.

Erythrocytes are formed early in life. Old and abnormal cells are destroyed.

Thrombocytes are formed in early life and as a compensatory mechanism. Effete cells are destroyed; increase after splenectomy.*

Reserve of blood elements. Part of the platelet pool exchange.

Iron is stored; participates in the iron metabolism.

Antibodies and opsonins are produced. Immune response mechanism may be reduced by its removal.

Leucocytes are controlled; elevation of their numbers occurs with removal of the gland. Phagocytosis-stimulating agent TUFTSIN produced.

Lymphocytes are stored early in the spleen. It participates in the reactive processes involving these cells. Both T and B lymphocytes are regulated.

Splenomegaly (1)

"MY PATH'S GREAT"

Note approximately three causes in each.

MYelosclerosis, myelogenous leukaemia, multiple myeloma.

Portal hypertension, pernicious anaemia, purpura.
Acholuric jaundice, abscess, anthrax.
Tropical: malaria, kala-azar, schistosomiasis.
Hodgkin's and other reticuloses.
Syphilis, septicaemia, Still's disease.

Glandular fever, Gaucher's disease, glycogen storage (von Gierke's).
Rupture, rickets, rats (leptospira icterohaemorrhagica).
Endocarditis (subacute), erythroblastosis fetalis, Egyptian splenomegaly (schistosomiasis and malaria).
Agranulocytosis, amyloidosis, aneurysm of the splenic artery.
Tumours (cysts), typhus, tuberculosis, typhoid and paratyphoid.

Splenomegaly (2): Shorter Version

"THAT CHIMP"

Typhoid, paratyphoid, typhus.
Hodgkin's and reticuloses.
Amyloid.
Tropical: kala-azar, malaria.

Cysts.
Haematological.
Infections.
Myeloid. Metabolic.
Portal hypertension.

Causes of Splenomegaly

"SPLENOMEGALICS"

Storage disease, Gaucher's.
Portal hypertension, pernicious anaemia, purpura.
Leukaemia and reticuloses, lymphatic and myeloid leukaemia.
Erythrocytes, spherocytosis, polycythaemia, erythroblastosis fetalis.
Neoplasms, cysts.
Operative or other injury (haematoma).
Malaria, myelosclerosis, multiple myeloma.
Endocarditis, subacute.
Glandular fever.
Amyloid, abscess, agranulocytosis, aneurysm of splenic artery.
Leishmaniasis.
Infections: brucellosis, anthrax, typhoid, paratyphoid, typhus, leptospira icterohaemorrhagica.
Cardiac failure.
Septicaemia, Still's disease, syphilis.

Causes of Hepatosplenomegaly

"PRISM"

Portal hypertension.
Reticuloses.
Infections: glandular fever.
Storage diseases: Gaucher's, amyloidosis.
Myeloproliferative and marrow diseases, e.g. pernicious anaemia, chronic myeloid leukaemia, sickle-cell anaemia.

Massive Enlargements of Spleen

FOUR Ms

Myeloid leukaemia.
Myelofibrosis.
Malaria.
Metabolic: Gaucher's syndrome.

Indications for Splenectomy

"TRACHEA"

Thrombocytopenic purpura.
Rupture.
Acholuric jaundice.
Cysts or tumours.
Hypersplenism. Hodgkin's disease to evaluate its stage.
Egyptian splenomegaly (schistosomiasis and malaria).
Aneurysm.

Complications of Splenectomy

"CLOSE THE SHOP"

Collapse of lung (pleura punctured).
Leucocytosis then lymphocytosis.
Obstructions, intestinal.
Stomach, acute dilatation.
Empyema of chest. Evisceration through wound.

Thrombocytosis, thromboses occur.*
Haematemesis.
Effusion of left pleural cavity.

Splenosis, sepsis.
Hiccup.
Osseous pain.
Pancreatitis.

Note: Also a-v fistula (rare).

CHAPTER 4

LIVER, GALL BLADDER AND BILE DUCTS

Functions of the Liver

A to P

Ammonia converted to urea. Amino acids and
   vitamin A stored.
Bile formed. Blood reserve. RBCs formed and
   destroyed. Vitamin B_{12} stored.
Carbohydrate metabolized. Conjugation of bilirubin.
   Coagulation factors.
Defence mechanism. Deamination and detoxification.
   Vitamin D stored.
Erythrocytes formed during fetal life.
Fat metabolized. Fibrinogen elaborated.
Glycogen metabolized. Glyconeogenesis. Glyco-
   genolysis.
Heat produced. Heparin and haematinic factor stored.
Ketone bodies formed from fat. Vitamin K formed and
   stored. Kuppfer's cells form globulin.
Liver failure results in fall in blood glucose level, then
   coma and death.
Mast cells produce the heparin.
Oestrogen and other hormones metabolized.
Prothrombin and plasma protein produced. Plasma
   phospholipids stored.

Mnemonics and Tactics

Enlargements of Liver

"TACTICS EARN M.D." is demonstrated.

Tumours.
   Innocent: haemangioma.
   Malignant: primary; cholangiomas, hepatic carcinomas, sarcomas.
   Secondaries.
Accident.
   Any blunt or penetrating injury leading to a haematoma.
   Postoperative cause such as portal pyaemia.
Congenital.
   Polycystic disease. Riedel's lobe enlargement.
Topical. Stone or stricture obstructing bile duct. Carcinoma of pancreas obstructing duct.
Tropical. Amoebiasis, hydatid cyst. Schistosomiasis, malaria, kala-azar.
Inflammations. Viral hepatitis, serum hepatitis, glandular fever, Weil's disease. Toxoplasmosis, tuberculosis.
Syphilis. Gummata.

Anaemias. Leukaemias.
Arteries. Aneurysm of hepatic artery.
Veins. Hepatic vein thrombosis.
Reticuloses. Hodgkin's etc.

Metabolic. Fatty change, cirrhosis, amyloid, haemochromatosis. Hurler's (gargoylism), glycogen storage disorder, Gaucher's disease.
Mechanical. Raised venous pressure, constrictive pericarditis, congestive heart failure.
Diet. Rickets, alcohol.
Drugs. Drugs and poisons.

Features of Hepatic Damage (1)

"SHEILA SHERLOCK"

Sex changes: in male, large breasts and small testes.
Hepatic fetor: sweet pungent odour of the breath.
External manifestations: spider naevi, liver palms, white nails.
Icterus, with or without associated itching.
Loss of weight.
Ascites and oedema.

Splenomegaly.
Haematological: low prothrombin, bleeding and sometimes thromboses.
Encephalopathy: toxic absorption of ammonia. May proceed from drowsiness to coma, delirium. Tremor.
Raised portal pressure may follow recovery.
Low-grade infection susceptibility.
Oesophageal varices and bleeding.
Clubbing of fingers (rare).
K and Na ions may be depressed in plasma.

With kind acknowledgement to Professor S. P. V. Sherlock, Royal Free Hospital. The author apologizes for the use of her name.

Mnemonics and Tactics

Features of Hepatic Damage (2)

"HEPATIC SIGNS"

Haematological due to vitamin K deficiencies, bleeding, purpura.
External manifestations: spider naevi, scratch marks, liver palms, purpura etc.
Portal hypertension, varices.
Ascites.
Tremor.
Itching.
Cachexia and clubbing.

Smell the breath.
Icterus.
Gynaecomastia and small testicles.
Neurological: encephalopathy and coma.
Splenomegaly.

Signs of Liver Damage in the Hands

Visible from a long distance

1. Liver flap.
2. Dupuytren's contracture.

Visible at the palms

1. Anaemia.
2. Thenar erythema.

Visible on the fingers

1. Clubbing.
2. Koilonychia.
3. Nail ridges.
4. Peripheral oedema.

Visible on the back of the hand

1. Spider naevi.
2. Jaundice.
3. Purpura and petechiae.
4. Boils susceptible to infection.

Causes of Cirrhosis

"CIRRHOSIS"

Congestive heart failure, chronic infection, e.g. ulcerative colitis, congenital, chemicals, carbon tetrachloride.
Infection: virus, idiopathic.
Retained iron or copper, haemochromatosis and Wilson's hepatolenticular degeneration respectively.
Reticulo-endothelial infiltrations, e.g. Gaucher's, amyloid, glycogen storage (von Gierke's).
Hanot's biliary cirrhosis (non-obstructive), hydatids.
Obstruction of bile ducts with or without infection.
Syphilis and starvation (inadequate diet).
Inebriation and idiopathic (50 per cent).
Schistosomiasis and flukes.

Incidence of malignant change in cirrhosis—10 per cent.

Contra-Indications to
Portal-Systemic Shunts

"HEAD C.I.A."

Hypo-albuminaemia.
Encephalopathy.
Aggressive hepatitis.
Diabetes mellitus.

Calcifications or partial thrombosis of portal vein.
Icterus.
Alcoholism.

Causes of Hepatic Calcification

"AGHAST"

Amoebic abscess.
Gumma.
Hydatid cyst, histoplasmosis, hepatoma.
Angioma.
Stones.
Tuberculosis.

Mnemonics and Tactics

Effects of Gall-Stones

"IMPACTS"

Impaction of stone: cystic, hepatic, common bile duct, at sphincter of Oddi, or ileum (gall-stone ileus). Mucus and pus may accumulate; function may be disturbed; perforation may follow impaction; pancreatitis may follow ductal outflow obstruction.

Malignant change may follow long-standing infection in gall bladder.

Pancreatitis may be associated with gall-stones.

Ascending cholangitis may occur with Charcot's intermittent fever. Abscesses may form in or behind liver.

Cholecystitis: acute, gangrenous, subacute or chronic with or without subsequent calcification.

Temperature, swinging, from empyema of gall bladder.

Strictures may form in common bile duct or sphincter of Oddi.

CHAPTER 5

PANCREAS

Surgical Complications of Diabetes

"NIKKOMAT"

Neuropathic, skeletal, trophic ulcers, Charcot joints.
Ischaemia, atherosclerosis, claudication, gangrene.
Kidney: carbuncle, pyelonephritis, pyonephritis, perinephric abscess.
Ketosis: acute abdomen, coma.
Ocular: retinopathy, cataract.
Multiple infections: boils, carbuncles, parotitis, poor wound healing.
Autonomic: diarrhoea, dysphagia.
Tuberculosis.

(*Note:* Correct spelling Nikkormat.)

Conditions Associated with Diabetes

"ACCEPT"

Acute pancreatitis.
Chronic pancreatitis.
Cushing's syndrome.
Excessive weight or steroids.
Pituitary tumours.
Thyrotoxicosis.

Causes of Acute Pancreatitis

"FATEMA'S BAGS"

Fibrocystic pancreas.
Ascariasis.
Trauma, include endoscopic cannulation, tumour and
    temperature (hypothermia).
Endocrine: parathyroid tumour.
Mumps or other viruses.
Atherosclerosis and hyperlipidaemia.
Sepsis: sialectasis.

Bile, regurgitation of infected; blockage of duct, e.g.
    catarrh.
Alcohol.
Gall-stones.
Steroids, azathioprine, opiates, thiazides, oestrogens
    etc.

And the bite of the Trinidad scorpion!

Features of Acute Pancreatitis (1)

"AMYLASES"

Acute prostrating pain, back and front.
Mid-abdominal and loin-staining.
Yellow with obstructive jaundice due to swollen
    pancreas or stone.
Lipase up.
Amylase up, calcium down.
Sugar may be present in the urine*. Small-bowel
    ileus.
Electrolytes lost; electrocardiographic changes.
Shock.

Features of Acute Pancreatitis (2)

"PANCREATITIS"

Pulseless with prostrating pain.*
Amylase* and lipase rise.
Nausea and copious vomiting.
Cyanosis. Calcium falls. Cullen and Grey Turner
   signs may appear (umbilicus and loin respectively).
Radiation of pain to back and shoulders.
   Right to left if duct becomes obstructed (rare).
Electrolytes are lost; profound shock* may ensue.
Abscess may form.
Tenderness rather than rigidity of the abdomen
   occurs. Rigidity follows the onset of peritonitis.
Icterus follows obstruction of biliary flow.
Tracings of the cardiogram are affected.
Ileus, particularly of the first loop of small bowel, is
   evident on plain X-ray.
Sugar may be found in the urine.*

Causes of Chronic Pancreatitis

"FASHIONS"

Fibrocystic disease.
Alcohol, atherosclerosis.
Syphilis.
Haemochromatosis, hyperparathyroidism.
Idiopathic.
Obstruction by stones or stenosis.
Neoplasm, slow-growing.
Steroids and other drugs.

Features of Chronic Pancreatitis

"MAIDS"

Malabsorption.
Abdominal pain.
Icterus.
Diabetes.
Steatorrhoea.

Features of Carcinoma of the Pancreas

"WINDBAG"

Widening of the duodenal loop.
Icterus, bile-duct occlusion by the primary or second-
aries.
Narrowing or encroachment on duodenal margin or
lumen.
Diabetes may be associated with it.
Back-ache.
Anorexia, abdominal pain and anaemia.
Gross loss of weight.

Causes of Elevated Amylase

"PROBLEM"

Pancreatitis and perforation of small intestine includ-
ing duodenal ulcer.
Renal infection.
Opiates.
Bowel obstruction. Bronchial carcinoma.
Loop stasis and liver disease.
Ectopic pregnancy.
Mumps and other salivary gland inflammation, and
macro-amylasaemia.

CHAPTER 6

PERITONEUM AND SMALL BOWEL

Causes of Ascites (1)

"CIRRHOSIS"

Congestive cardiac failure, constrictive pericarditis.
Idiopathic.
Renal failure.
Rotations: strangulation.
Hepatic cirrhosis, hypoproteinaemia, hypertension
  (portal), hypothyroidism.
Ovarian tumours: pseudomyxoma peritonei, Meigs'
  syndrome.
Schistosomiasis, starvation.
Infection: tuberculosis, inflammations, acute
  pancreatitis, infarcts, etc.
Secondaries.

Causes of Ascites (2)

"HORRID ITCH"

Hepatic: hypertension (portal), cirrhosis.
Ovarian: pseudomyxoma peritonei, Meigs' syndrome.
Renal failure.
Rotations.
Idiopathic.
Diet: kwashiorkor, starvation.

Inflammatory: acute pancreatitis, infection, tuber-
culosis, infarct.
Tumours: secondaries.
Cardiac failure, constrictive pericarditis.
Hypoproteinaemia.

Causes of Ascites (3)

"ASCITES"

Acid-fast infection (tuberculosis).
Starvation, kwashiorkor.
Cardiac causes and cirrhosis.
Inflammation: pancreatitis, peritonitis.
Tumours: secondaries, ovarian (Meigs' syndrome).
Excess loss of protein: nephroses, protein-losing
enteropathy, malabsorption.
Strangulation.

Causes of Venous Thrombosis and Mesenteric Arterial Embolus or Thrombosis

"A BAD PASS"

Venous Thrombosis

Accident.

Buerger's disease.
Appendicitis, diverticulitis.
Dehydration.

Portal hypertension.
Anaemia.
Splenectomy (rise in platelets).
Strangulation.

Mesenteric Arterial Embolus or Thrombosis

Atrial fibrillation (80 per cent).

Bacterial endocarditis.
Arteriosclerosis.
Dissecting aneurysm.

Polyarteritis nodosa.
Abdominal saccular aneurysm, pressure effects or emboli.
Strangulation, e.g. volvulus, hernia.
Sepsis: intra-abdominal, eg. appendicitis.

Causes of Blood-Stained Fluid
in Peritoneal Cavity

FOUR Ss

Sweetbread: pancreatitis, acute.
Secondaries.
Strangulations, herniae, ovaries.
Stoppage of blood flow. Mesenteric emboli or
    thrombosis.

or

"PISS"

Pancreatitis.
Infarction.
Strangulation.
Secondaries.

Causes of Peritonitis

"HIPPOCRATES"

Haemorrhagic, e.g. pancreatitis.

Infection of the peritoneum, pneumoccocal, tuberculosis.

Perforation: peptic ulcer, diverticulitis, carcinoma, ulcerative colitis, etc.

Postoperative: leaking anastomosis, swab or FB left in.

Occlusion of mesenteric vessels leading to gangrene.

Congenital: perforated meconium ileus, volvulus etc.

Rupture by accident or FB.

Acute appendicitis.

Typhoid.

Empyema of gall bladder with spreading infection.

Strangulations, including external herniae.

Causes of Internal and External Fistulae
(Abdominal Area)

"TACTICS"

Tumours. Malignant tumours of stomach, colon, small bowel (rare), bladder, cervix.

Accident. Penetrating injuries, FBs.

Post-irradiation.

Postoperative. Leaking anastomosis, retained swab or FB.

Congenital. Anorectal anomalies, ectopia vesicae, urachus etc., patent Meckel's.

Topical. Strangulated hernia with perforation. Post-appendicectomy. Peptic ulcer with gastro-jejunocolic fistula. Ileostomy (therapeutic).

Tropical. Typhoid, amoebiasis.

Inflammation. Tuberculosis, Crohn's, ulcerative colitis, actinomycosis, lymphogranuloma venereum.

Persistence of Fistula

"FISTULA"

FB present.
Irradiated area.
Syphilis: sequestrum.
Tumour, tuberculosis.
Unable to transmit faeces or urine through conduit
    due to presence of stricture.*
Lining development. Mucosa may grow and line tube.
Actinomycosis.

Congenital Abnormalities of Bowel

"MIGRAINES"

Meckel and meconium ileus.
Imperforate or absent anus with or without a fistula.
Grossly high caecum.
Reversed appendix, thoracic and abdominal viscera,
    situs inversus viscerum.
Atresia and annular pancreas.
Ischaemia of bowel and strictures.
Neonatal volvulus.
Exomphalos.
Stenosis of pylorus (hypertrophic), or diaphragm at
    level of duodenum.

Intestinal Obstruction in the Newborn

The A.B.C.D.E.F. of Intestinal Obstruction

Alkalosis and shock follows the vomiting, which may or may not contain bile.

Blood may be present in the stools or vomitus with intestinal necrosis, e.g. intussusceptions, rotations.

Constipation may follow the passage of a few stools.
  Cyanosis occurs with diaphragmatic hernia.
  Choking or coughing with oesophageal atresia.

Distension varies with the height of the obstruction and impairs diaphragmatic breathing.

Electrolyte changes require careful monitoring.

Farber's test using gentian violet to identify swallowed epithelial skin cells.

Differential Diagnosis from above downwards.

Head: intracranial lesions.

Oesophagus and diaphragm: atresias and herniae.

Stomach: volvulus and meconium gastritis.

Pylorus: hypertrophic stenosis.

Duodenum and pancreas: atresia, bands, annular pancreas, duodenal diaphragm.

Small bowel: volvulus, intussusception, meconium ileus, Meckel anomalies, herniae internal and external.

Colon and rectum: atresia with or without fistulae, Hirschsprung's disease.

Causes of Intestinal Obstruction

"HERNIA"

Hernia: external or internal, strangulated or non-strangulated.
Embolism, mesenteric.
Regional ileitis.
Neoplasm: innocent or malignant, primary or secondary.
Ileus due to infection, appendicitis, diverticulitis, and intussusception.
Adhesions: congenital or acquired. Postoperative.

Note: Causes can be sought by utilizing "TACTICS".

Classification of Causes of Intestinal Obstruction

"SPLASH"

Specific causes: tumours, adhesions, inflammations.
Partial or complete, open- or closed-loop.
Level: above or below a competent or incompetent
   ileocaecal valve.
Adynamic or dynamic, arterial or venous obstruction.
Strangulation or non-strangulation.
Herniae.*

Causes of Stricture of Small Bowel

"ACCIDENT"

Acid-fast infection.
Crohn's disease.
Congenital: atresia.
Ischaemia.
Drugs: potassium chloride, etc.
Enteric fever.
Neoplasia: carcinoma, carcinoids, sarcomata,
   secondaries.
Trauma: postoperative complications, ileostomy
   stoma.

Causes of Paralytic Ileus

FIVE Ps and FIVE Rs

Postoperative.
Peritonitis.
Pelvic and spinal fractures (plaster of Paris jacket).
Potassium low.
Parturition.

Renal failure.
Renal colic.
Retroperitoneal haemorrhage.
Retroperitoneal infection.
Raised blood sugar — diabetes.

Causes of Diarrhoea (1)

"UNFORMED STOOLS"

Uraemia, ulcerative colitis, Crohn's disease.
Nervous: anxiety, irritable colon.
Fistula and faecal impaction.
Obstruction of bile duct.
Resection of bowel, stomach, vagus.
Malignancy: includes multiple polyposis, an innocent
    condition.
Endocrine: thyrotoxicosis, carcinoids, Zollinger-
    Ellison syndrome.
Diverticulitis and drugs.

Sprue.
Tropical: amoebiasis, worms.
Obstructed pancreatic ducts, pancreatitis.
Obstruction of bowel, strictures, gall-stone, ileus.
Loop (stagnant-loop syndrome).
Specific infections: typhoid, paratyphoid, salmonella,
    etc.

Causes of Diarrhoea (2)

"PASS BIG DUTCH CAP"

Pancreatic tumours or dysfunction.
Anxiety states. Amyloid disease.
Subacute and chronic intestinal obstruction.
Stricture, sprue, steatorrhoea.

Bacteria: salmonella, tuberculosis, typhoid, typhus,
    paratyphoid, shigella, *E. coli*, cholera, staphylococ-
    cal enterocolitis.
Impacted faeces. Ischaemic colitis.
Gastrocolic fistula, gastro-enterostomy and vagotomy.

Drugs: digitalis, antibiotics, diverticulitis. Poisons:
    lead, mushrooms.
Ulcerative colitis and uraemia.
Tumours and thyrotoxicosis.
Carcinoid tumours, closed-loop syndrome.
Hernia (Richter), hurry, HCl lack, hemicolectomy (R).

Crohn's or coeliac disease.
Amoebiasis.
Pelvic abscess, peritonitis in children, parasites.

See causes of malabsorption, page 79.

Also try "TACTICS".

Causes of Constipation

"CONSTIPATED"

Congenital: Hirschsprung's Disease.
Obstruction.
Neoplasms.
Stricture as in Crohn's, following ischaemia; post-operative.
Topical: painful piles or fissure.
Impacted faeces.
Prolapse of the rectum.
Anorexia and depression.
Temperature high, dehydration results.
Endocrine: hypothyroidism, hyperparathyroidism.
Diet, diverticulitis and drugs.

Blind- or Stagnant-Loop Syndrome

"SALAD"

Steatorrhoea.
Anaemia.
Loss of weight.
Abdominal pains.
Deficiencies of vitamins.

Mnemonics and Tactics

Causes of Blood in Stool (1)

Use "TACTICS" etc.

Tumours. Innocent: adenomatous polyps, villous papillomas, tubulo-villous lesions, multiple polyposis, angiomata. Malignant: lesions from oesophagus to anus, particularly of colon.

Accident. Blunt penetrating wounds, foreign body such as chicken bone. X-ray damage leading to proctitis or enteritis. Postoperative after any operation on alimentary tract, particularly haemorrhoidectomy (1 per cent). Swallowed blood.

Tropical. Amoebiasis.

Topical. Piles, fissure, faecal impaction. Peptic ulcer of oesophagus, stomach, duodenum, jejunum, adjacent to Meckel's diverticulum. Diverticulitis.

Inflammation. Proctocolitis from any cause, gonococcal, tuberculous, or dysenteric. Typhoid.

Collagen. Periarteritis with lesions in bowel.

Anaemias. Henoch or Schönlein purpuras. Haemophilia. Afibrinogen states. Veins. Piles may be due to portal hypertension. Arterial embolus or thrombosis. Venous thrombosis.

Metabolic disease. Uraemia.

Mechanical. Volvulus, intussusception.

Drugs. Cytotoxic, aspirin, Indocid, potassium — ulceration occurs.

Gertrude. Gynaecological, endometriosis.

Causes of Blood in Stool (2)

"PICTURE PARADES"

Peptic ulcer.

Intussusception.

Carcinoma: oesophagus, stomach, pancreas, duodenum (very rare), small bowel (rare), colon,
rectum, anal canal, anus.

Thrombosis, arterial or venous.

Ulcerative colitis, Crohn's.

Rotations, volvulus. Strangulated hernia.

Endometriosis.

Polyposis coli. Polyps.

Accidents: penetrating lesions, postoperative.

Rectal lesions: piles, fissure.

Anaemias, anticoagulants.

Diverticulitis, Meckel's diverticulum with peptic
ulceration.

Entamoeba histolytica, enteritis, enteric fever.

Swallowed blood.

Causes of Massive Haemorrhage

"RACED"

Ruptured aneurysm (rare).

Amoebic colitis.

Colitis, ulcerative.

Enteric fever.

Diverticulitis.

Mnemonics and Tactics

Causes of Malabsorption

Defective absorption of essential food factors.

"MALABSORPTION"

Metabolic: disaccharidase deficiency, Hartnup disease.

Acid-fast (tuberculosis), infection of bowel.

Liver disease: lipodystrophy (Whipple's disease).

Atherosclerosis: ischaemic changes.

Blind-loop syndrome, fistulae, gastrojejunocolic fistula.

Systemic sclerosis.

Obstruction: stricture of small bowel.

Resection: stomach or intestine.

Pancreas, fibrocystic disease, pancreatitis.

Tropical: sprue, tapeworms.

Idiopathic steatorrhoea. Coeliac syndrome. Inflammation of bowel (Crohn's disease).

Obstruction of bile ducts.

Neoplasia: multiple polyps (or cysts).

Features of Steatorrhoea

"STEATORRHOEA"

Serum iron low.
Tetany.
Electrocardiogram changes due to low K, Mg and Ca.
Abdominal distension.
Thrombotest prolonged. Malabsorption of vitamin K
   and other fat-soluble vitamins.
Offensive stools. Toilet flushing.
Radiology shows osteomalacia.
Ravenous appetite or anorexia may be present.
Hypoproteinaemia occurs.
Oedema may develop due to loss of protein.
Endocrine changes: secondary hyperparathyroidism
   may occur.
Anaemia, either macro- or microcytic in form, due to
   fall in B_{12}, folate or Fe.

Meckel's Diverticulum

TWOs

Two per cent of people, two feet from ileocaecal valve *approximately,* two inches long.

Complications of Meckel's Diverticulum

SEVEN Ps

Peptic ulceration of adjacent mucosa and melaena.
Perforation and general peritonitis.
Pain: colicky with intussusception.
Pink: raspberry tumour at umbilicus.
Patent vitello-intestinal duct with or without ductal stenosis.
Persisting band with strangulations or cysts anywhere along the track.
Persistent umbilical discharge may contain hydrochloric acid.

Classification of Small-Bowel Tumours

Try routine as in "TACTICS"

(*Note:* duodenum is included in small-bowel tumours.*)

Innocent. Polyps, adenomata, haemangioma.
Malignant. Primary: include ampullary tumours. Secondary: hormone-producing carcinoids.
Reticuloses. Lymphosarcoma etc.
Gynaecology. Endometrioma.
Congenital. Pancreatic rests.
And syndromes. See below.

Peutz-Jegher: Polyposis of small bowel and "dog's mouth" (pigmentation).
Gardner's syndrome: Duodenal polyps, etc.

Intussusception in Infants

A.B.C.D.E.F.

Abdominal or anal "sausage".
Blood *per rectum** (red-currant jelly). Barium enema is useful.
Colic. Babies draw up their legs.
Distension, dehydration and shock.
Emesis. Equal incidence.
Facies pale.

Pale* off his food and very still,
Means the child is bloody ill.

Mucoviscidosis (1)

"THAT MUCOVISCIDOSIS"

Tense distended abdomen.
Hydrogen peroxide for washing out bowel.
Autosomal recessive gene responsible.
Trypsin lack in vomitus: it has no lytic effect on X-ray film.

Meconium thick and obstructive.
Ulceration of the duodenum may occur in association with this condition.
Cystic and fibrotic changes occasionally in cervix and prostate.
Obstruction of air passages: atelectasis, bronchiectasis, bronchitis, etc.
Viscidity of mucus increases.
Infection of mucus in lungs with staphylococci.
Secretion of all glands may be affected.
Cough.
Ileus.
Dilated ducts in pancreas.
Obstruction of bowel.
Stenosis of pancreatic duct may be present.
Involvement of liver may go on to cirrhosis.
Sodium chloride excess in sweat, loss leads to heat sensitivity.

Mucoviscidosis (2)

"BAD SPICES"

Biliary cirrhosis.
Appetite voracious.
Distended abdomen.

Secondary infection. Sticky mucus. Stricture.
Pancreatitis. Perforation.
Intestinal obstruction.
Chest involvement.
Excess salt in sweat. Eye changes.
Steatorrhoea.

Clinical Picture of Ileus

"DANCER"

Distension.
Absent bowel sounds.
Nausea, vomiting, faecal vomiting.
Constipation: absolute.
Electrolytes lost; shock ensues.
Rising pulse, falling blood pressure.

Carcinoid Syndrome

"CARCINOIDS"

Cyanosis due to cor pulmonale.

Asthma due to the stimulation of the smooth muscle by serotonin. Alcohol may precipitate the attack.

Rubor, attacks of flushing.

Cor pulmonale.

Incompetent tricuspid and pulmonary valves due to endocardial fibrosis.

Noisy abdomen due to over-activity.

Oedema.

Indoles in the urine, 5,hydroxy-indole acetic acid.

Diarrhoea. (*Note:* Detoxification occurs in the liver and lungs.)

Smooth muscle is stimulated by the secretion. The effects are only produced by secondaries in or beyond the liver.

An alternative word is "FACADES"

Flushing.

Asthma.

Cor pulmonale.

Ascites.

Diarrhoea.

Endocardial fibrosis. Ehrlich's reagent for the urine test.

Secondaries in or beyond the liver produce the effects.

Crohn's Disease (1)

Some features of the disease.

"CROHN'S"

Cobblestones on X-ray.
Rectal involvement with abscesses or fistulae may occur.
Obstructions of bowel.
Hyperplasia of mesenteric lymph glands.
Narrowing of ileum produces Kantor's string sign.
Skip lesions, steatorrhoea, sarcoid foci (70 per cent).

Features of Crohn's Disease (2)

Further features, the majority of which are indications for operation:

"SPASMODIC"

Stricture.
Perforation.
Acute appendicitis simulated.
Sepsis, abscess.
Mass.
Obstructions.
Deficiencies: vitamin B_{12}, etc.
Internal and external fistulae.
Cachexia.

CHAPTER 7

COLON, RECTUM AND ANAL CANAL

Congenital Anomalies of Colon

"HEADS"

Hirschprung's disease.
Enterogenous cysts.
Atresia or absence of colon.
Double-barrelled colon.
Small (micro-) colon.

Some Features of Hirschprung's Disease

A.B.C.D.E.F.

Anus is normal; no soiling. Aganglionic segment is the cause.
Borborygmi are abnormal due to obstruction. Biopsy shows absence of ganglion cells.
Constipation may soon become complete and necessitate a defunctioning colostomy.
Distension of the abdomen is marked.
Empty rectum is found on digital examination.
Familial.

Features of Ulcerative Colitis

"ULCERATIVE COLITIS"

Ulcers: leg, gut and mouth.
Low abdominal pain.
Carcinomatous change.
Emaciation.
"Rotting" of liver (cirrhosis).
Anaemia, arthritis, amyloid.
Toxic dilatation.
Infections, low state of patient.
Vitamin deficiencies.
Erosion of bowel wall and perforation.

Clubbing.
Obstructions.
Loss of K and water.
Iridocyclitis, and toxic manifestations, pyodermia, erythema nodosum, urticaria,
Tracks, fistulae.
Iatrogenic, from steroids, blood transfusion.
Strictures.

Ulcerative Colitis: Indications for Operation

"MAP OF PARIS"

Malignant change present or suspected.
Acute colonic dilatation or acute fulminant disease.
Perforation.

Over 8 or 10 years, to avoid chance of malignant change.
Fistula internal.

Pseudopolypotic state.
Anaemia: acute bleeding or chronic blood loss, particularly rare blood group.
Rectal disease with fistulae, stenoses, recurrent abscesses.
Iridocyclitis and other toxic manifestations, pyoderma, multiple arthritis etc.
Stricture.

Mnemonics and Tactics

Complications of Colostomies

"COLOSTOMIES"

Contracture or stricture. (*Note:* Mucocutaneous
   approximation by suture avoids it.)
Obstruction in the lateral space.
Leaks: blood or faeces.
Obstruction due to kinking or herniation of bowel
   around colostomy.
Slips in.
Torsion.
Obstruction due to faecal impaction.
Mental effects.
Infection, wound or peritoneum.
Excoriation around the colostomy, particularly if right
   colon is utilized.
Slips out. Prolapse occurs with straining.

Causes of Pruritus Ani (1)

"PIGS"

Psychogenic.

Infection and allergy, scabies, fungi, worms, Candida.

General: diabetes mellitus, Hodgkin's disease, jaundice.

Soggy skin, due to sweating or abnormal mucus or purulent discharge, e.g. piles, prolapse, fistulae, Crohn's disease, diverticulitis, etc.

Causes of Pruritus Ani (2)

Classification — Anatomical

Anal canal. Haemorrhoids, fissure, fistulae, tumours, prolapse, worms.

Rectum. Proctitis, proctocolitis, including Crohn's disease.

Bowel. Amoebiasis, diverticulitis, fistulae.

Urethra. Incontinence, urethritis.

Vagina. Cervicitis, Trichomonas, Candida.

Skin: general. Diabetes, Hodgkin's disease, jaundice, etc.

Skin: perianal. Mycotic, allergy, poor hygiene, sweating, irritation by liquid paraffin, neurosis, hypersensitivity, parasites, etc.

"PRURITUS ANI"

Prolapse: uterus, vagina, rectum.
Rectal causes, including proctitis, proctocolitis, Crohn's disease.
Urethral and vaginal causes, including urethritis, incontinence, cervicitis, Trichomonas, Candida.
Recumbency: postoperative, with poor hygiene.
Infection: bacteria, fungi, fleas, pediculosis.
Tropical: amoebiasis, lymphogranuloma venereum.
Unctions (ointments), drugs leading to allergy.
Systemic causes: diabetes, Hodgkin's disease, jaundice, psoriasis, etc.

Anal causes: piles, chronic fissure, polyps, fistulae, mucous discharge.
Nervous: psychological.
Intestinal: diverticulitis, neoplasia.

Tumours of Rectum and Anus

Innocent

"PALE"

Papilloma, villous.
Adenomata, including tubular variety.
Lymphoma, lipoma.
Endometrioma.

Malignant

"RASCAL"

Rodent ulcer of anal margin.
Adenocarcinoma.
Squamous cell carcinoma.
Carcinoid tumour.
Amelanotic or melanotic melanoma.
Lymphosarcoma.

Carcinoma of the Rectum: Clinical Features

"CA. RECTUMS"

Change in bowel habit.
Anaemia and bleeding: beware of associated piles.*

Rectal disease: ulcerative colitis, polyposis. Adenomatous polyps and villous papillomas.
Enlarging abdomen.
Cachexia. Cervical glands on the left above the clavicle (rare).
Tenesmus and pain.
Ulcer and unsatisfied defaecation.
Mucus may be blood-stained.
Spurious diarrhoea and sensation of "something being there".

Causes of Anorectal and Colonic Strictures

SIX Is

Inflammation: Crohn's, colitis, lymphogranuloma, amoebiasis, diverticulitis, tuberculosis.

Injury: post-haemorrhoidectomy, following imperfect bowel anastomoses postoperative.

Irradiation.

Inherited: anorectal atresia.

Infiltrating neoplasm: primary or secondary.

Ischaemia is added for colon strictures.

Note: Spasm caused by "fissure", and senile anal stenosis.

Causes of Prolapse of Rectum

"PROLAPSES"

Psychotics.
Rectal lesions, worms and polyps in children.
Old age.
Labour damage to puborectalis.
Abnormal habits, prolonged sitting and straining at
  stool.
Piles, may develop into prolapse.
Spinal lesions.
Emaciation.
Stricture of urethra with straining.

Causes of Mass in Rectum

"PRACTICAL"

Prostrate: normal, innocent or malignant. Prostatic abscess.

Reticuloses: Hodgkin's disease, etc. Retroverted uterus.

Abscess: pelvic, perianal, or perirectal.

Cervix: normal or diseased.

Tumour of rectum: e.g. carcinoma, or sacral chordoma, or mass in the rectovesical pouch or pouch of Douglas.

Impacted faeces.

Crohn's disease.

Amoebiasis.

Lymphogranuloma forming inflammatory mass. Loose body.

Causes of Anal Canal Pain

It makes you "FAINT"

Fissure, fugax proctalgia.

Acute diarrhoea, proctitis with excoriation.

Ischiorectal abscess. Infection.

Neoplasm, ulcerated.

Thrombosed piles.

CHAPTER 8

APPENDIX

Mass in Right Iliac Fossa (1)

"RIGHT ILIAC FOSSA"

Renal or retroperitoneal mass (ureter).
Intussusception.
Gynaecological causes.
Hernia, incisional, may be irreducible.
Terminal ileitis (Crohn's disease), undescended
   testicle.

Inferior epigastric bleed with haematoma.
Lymph-gland enlargements: iliac or mesenteric.
Iliac artery aneurysm, ileocaecal tuberculosis.
Appendix abscess or mass.*
Carcinoma or tumours of right colon,* appendix, small
   bowel.

From above, liver, gall bladder.
Obstructed bowel loop, volvulus, faecal mass.
Spleen (rare).
Spinal sepsis, psoas abscess.
Amoebiasis.

Mass in Right Iliac Fossa (2)

1. Appendix abscess or mass: Crohn's disease, ileocaecal tuberculosis (rare). Actinomycosis (rare). Glands.
2. Tumours: innocent or malignant, primary or secondary, e.g. colon, appendix, small bowel.
3. From above: liver, gall bladder, kidney.
4. From below: ovary, undescended testicle, Fallopian tube, uterus, bladder or its diverticulum.
5. From behind: psoas abscess, glands, aneurysm, and tumours.
6. From left: intussusception, and spleen and pelvic colon.
7. From in front: herniae, haematoma, lipoma.
8. From outside ("overseas"): amoebiasis, worms.

Differential Diagnosis of Pain in Right Side of Abdomen

"ACUTE APPENDICITIS"

Acute pancreatitis, acute hepatitis (incubating).
Cholecystitis. Chest infection in children.
Ureteric colic.
Torsion of ovarian cyst.
Ectopic pregnancy. Embolus, mesenteric artery.

Adenitis, mesenteric* or iliac.
Perforation: duodenum, salpinx or ovarian follicle.
Pneumonia (diaphragmatic pleurisy), pneumococcal peritonitis, pregnancy.
Enterocolitis. Ear: otitis media in children.
Neoplasm: caecum, right colon, appendix ileum, neurosis.
Diabetes: pre-coma.
Intestinal obstruction, or constipation, inferior epigastric vessels rupture.
Coronary thrombosis.
Ileitis: Crohn's disease. Intestinal obstruction.
Tabetic crisis.
Inflammation, urinary tract: pyelocystitis.*
Salpingitis, shingles.

Complications of Appendicitis and Appendicectomy

Variables: Depends on site, spread of infection, perforation, gangrene of the appendix, and other complications.

Example: Appendicitis in the right iliac fossa.

1. At site: abscess, mass (omentum) with loops of adherent bowel, intestinal obstructions, released faecolith, swab left in.
2. Ascending infection: portal pyaemia, subphrenic abscess.
3. Descending: pelvic abscess, cystitis, vesico-intestinal fistula, false diverticulum of bladder, tubo-ovarian mass, Fallopian-tube damage.
4. Spreading backwards: cellulitis, abscess sited retroperitoneally, iliac-vein thrombosis, psoas spasm.
5. Spreading forwards: mass, abscess, sinus, fistula.
6. Spreading medially: general peritonitis, ileus, adhesions, obstructions.

Summary of Obstructive Appendicitis in the child

Central colicky pain, copious vomiting, and a very sick child.

CHAPTER 9

BREAST AND ANTERIOR ABDOMINAL WALL

Causes of Gynaecomastia (1)

"GYNAECOMASTIA"

Gynaecological and other drugs: oestrogens, digitalis, etc.
Young males:* neonatal and during puberty.
Neoplasms: lung and testicle.
Albright's syndrome.
Excessive or reduced thyroid activity.
Cirrhosis.
Orchitis following mumps.
Malnutrition.
Adrenocortical tumours.
Sex: hermaphrodite, Klinefelter's syndrome.
Traumatic paraplegia.
Iodine, radioactive.
Adenoma (chromophobe) of pituitary. Acromegaly (eosinophilic).

Causes of Gynaecomastia (2)

"ASKANCE AT HIM"

Acromegaly.
Sex hormones.
Klinefelter's syndrome.
Albright's syndrome.
Neoplasm: lung carcinoma.
Cirrhosis.
Endocrine (other): hyperthyroidism, hypothyroidism,
    pituitary adenoma, adrenal tumours.

Amphetamine, digitalis, radio-iodine and other drugs.
    Adolescence.
Testicular tumours.

Hermaphrodites and pseudohermaphrodites.
Injury to spinal cord, paraplegia.
Malnutrition.

Umbilical Fistulae

Thick yellow pus: peritonitis.

Thin yellowish pus: tuberculosis.

Urine due to patent urachus.

Mucus due to vestigial vitello-intestinal duct.

Bile-stained or bile.

Faecal due to patent vitello-intestinal duct, or Crohn's disease or (malignant) bowel fistula.

Blood from endometriosis or ectopic gastric mucosa in vitello-intestinal anomaly.

Fluid showing acid reactions, from ectopic gastric mucosa.

Fibro-Adenosis of Breast

Five Ways of Presentation

Clinically
1. As large or multiple cysts.
2. Localized mass or masses in breast.
3. Single or bilateral breast pain.
4. Discharge from nipple.
5. Mastitis, tender with hyperaemia.

Microscopically
1. Adenosis may lead to fibro-adenosis.
2. Epitheliosis may be followed by malignant change.
3. Fibrosis.
4. Cystosis.
5. Lymphocytic infiltration.

Acute Inflammation of the Breast

Five Acute Inflammations
1. Hormonal in newborn and adolescence.
2. Acute infections complicating lactation.
3. Traumatic due to chafing.
4. Infection of the glands of Montgomery.
5. Mumps.

Traumatic Fat Necrosis

Five Points
1. Follows injury to fatty tissues, e.g. breast, buttock or leg.
2. May be preceded by bruising.
3. Hard, due to fibrosis and chalk deposits.
4. Attached to skin, may have overlying peau d'orange.
5. Becomes smaller as time elapses.*

Chronic Abscesses of Breast

Five Varieties
1. Pyogenic.
2. Tuberculous (rare).
3. Actinomycosis (rare).
4. Gummatous (rare).
5. Secondary to retromammary infection (rare).

Tuberculosis of Breast

Five Origins
1. Rib and spine.
2. Mediastinal cervical or axillary glands.
3. Pleura and lung.
4. Blood-borne.
5. Complicating tuberculous lesion of skin.

Note: Tuberculosis of breast is very rare.

Cysts of Breast

Five Cysts of Breast
1. Cyst of fibro-adenosis.
2. Galactocele appears during lactation.
3. Retention cyst of glands of Montgomery.
4. Cystic changes in tumours.
5. Hydatid cysts.

Five Discharges from Nipple
1. Milky.
2. Brownish-yellow or green of chronic mastitis.
3. Purulent.
4. Blood-stained fluid.
5. Serous: early pregnancy.

Causes of Blood-Stained Discharge from Nipple

Five Causes
1. Paget's disease of nipple.
2. Eczema of nipple.
3. Duct papilloma.
4. Intradermal carcinoma.
5. Carcinoma involving ductal system.

Tuberculous Infections

Five Varieties
1. Discharging sinus.
2. Nodule.
3. Diffuse caseation: multiple abscesses and ulcers.
4. Sclerosing variety.
5. Obliterating mastitis. Ducts are obliterated.

Carcinoma of Breast

Varieties of pathology

"APPLES"

Atrophic scirrhous (adenocarcinoma).
Papillary.
Paget's disease of the nipple.
Lactational: mastitis carcinomatosis.
Encephaloid.
Scirrhous.

Breast

Physical signs relating to nipple:

FIVE Ds

Discharge.
Depression or inversion.
Discoloration: pregnancy.
Dermatological changes: Paget's disease.
Deviation: compare opposite side.

Differentiation of Lumps in the Breast

Distinguish by adherence to the skin:

Five Lumps Attached to the Skin
1. Carcinoma.
2. Fat necrosis. Follows an injury and becomes smaller.
3. Abscess pyogenic, tuberculosis, may persist as fistula.
4. Resolving haematoma.
5. Plasma cell mastitis.

Five Lumps Unattached to the Skin
1. Carcinoma.
2. Cysts, fibro-adenosis.
3. Fibro-adenoma, pericanalicular and intra-canalicular.
4. Duct papilloma (premalignant).
5. Other innocent tumours: lipoma, angioma, etc.

Mnemonics and Tactics

Features and Causes of Abdominal Dehiscence

"ABDOMINAL DEHISCENCE"

Anaemia.
Blood in wound.
Defective technique.
Obstruction of bowel.*
Metabolic: uraemia, diabetes.
Infection of wound.
Nutrition: starvation.
Anaesthetist: pharyngeal suction with coughing and straining may cause rupture.
Location: upper abdominal incisions most likely to rupture.

Distension of bowel, e.g. ileus or obstruction.
Enlarged bladder.
Hypoprotinaemia.
Infection: intraperitoneal.
Steroids.
Chronic cough.*
Eight to ten days is critical time.
Neoplasm with cachexia.*
C vitamin deficiency.
Enzyme leakage: pancreatitis.

Large Abdomen

NINE Fs

Fat.
Faeces.
Flatus.
Fluid.
Full bladder.
Fibroid.
Fetus.
False pregnancy.
Firm mass: kidney, liver, spleen, ovary etc.

Lumps in Groin

"SAPHENA"

Saphena varix.
Aneurysm of femoral artery.
Psoas abscess.
Hernia and hydrocele of cord.
Ectopic testis.
Nodes, lymph.
Abscess.

CHAPTER 10

HERNIAE Etc

Swellings in the Groins

Five Cysts
Herniae, cyst of cord.
Saphena varix.
Psoas abscess (rare).
Cystic hygroma (rare).
Baker's cyst of hip joint. Femoral artery pushed
    forward resembles an aneurysm (rare). Aneurysm.

Five Solid Lumps
Irreducible herniae.
Infected glands.
Tumour-involved glands, secondaries or reticuloses.
Ectopic testis.
Connective tissue tumours, lipoma etc.

Definition of strangulated hernia
Tense tender lump with vomiting.

Examination of Hernia

"STIC"

Stand patient up.
Testicles: feel both.
Internal ring half an inch above midinguinal point
   controls indirect hernia.
Cough (expansile): test both. Cause* is sought.

Causes of Herniae

"HERNIA CAUSE"

Heavy lifting.
Excessive coughing.
Raised intra-abdominal pressure.
Nerve damage as occurs in Battle's incision for
    appendicectomy.
Infection following first repair.
Ageing.

Congenital defect. sac.
Anal stricture.
Urethral stricture.
Straining due to constipation.
Excessively fat.

CHAPTER 11

KIDNEYS, URETERS, ADRENALS AND BLADDER

Tests for Kidney Disease

"PARADISE"

Perirenal air insufflation.
Arteriogram, arterial samples for analysis.
Renal biopsy, retrograde pyelogram.
Aspiration, cysts.
Determination of blood pressure and blood
    constituents.
Intravenous pyelogram, tomograms, cine radiography.
Straight X-ray. Sonic studies.
Evaluate function of one or both kidneys. Examine
    urine fully.

Causes of Nephrocalcinosis

"MEDICINES"

Multiple myeloma.
Endocrine: hyperparathyroidism, Cushing's syndrome.
D: excess vitamin D.
Immobilization and osteoporosis.
Chronic pyelonephritis.
Interference with pH: renal tubular acidosis.
Necrosis of renal papilla.
Excessive steroid therapy.
Sarcoidosis; secondaries, osteolytic; sponge medullary kidney.

Causes of Localized Nephrocalcinosis

"CHAT M.P."

Cyst.
Hydatid.
Acid-fast infection.
Tumour: hypernephroma.

Medullary sponge kidney.
Papillary necrosis.

Causes of Recurrent Urinary Stones

"DISEASED"

Diet: too much vitamin D and calcium (alkalis);
   too little vitamin A and water.
Infection: particularly the urea-splitters.
Stasis: above stricture.
Endocrine: parathyroid tumours, Cushing's syndrome.
Abnormal amounts or constituents: cystine indigo
   xanthine (CIX) etc., uric acid, oxalate, hyper-
   oxaluria.
Sarcoidosis.
Excess calcium in urine.
Decubitus: recumbency in bed, and poor drainage.

Uraemia

ELEVEN Ds

Dirty face, tongue, mouth, breath and dirty taste in mouth.

Drowsiness, disorientation, delirium.

Dysphagia, dyspepsia, distension, diminished bowel sounds and diarrhoea, possibly a dilated full bladder.

Dermatological changes: dry skin, pruritus, urea frost, lax if dehydrated.

Dyspnoea, distressing "Kussmaul" (gasping) breathing.

Dimness of vision, nipping, haemorrhages, papill-oedema.

Demyelinization and degeneration of nerves.

Decalcification and dystrophy of bones; patients become resistant to vitamin D, and calcium absorption falls.

Dyscrasias of blood; bleeding from gums, purpura.

Depletion of sodium due to vomiting and polyuria.

Digitalis tolerance is reduced.

Note: This list is not comprehensive.

Causes of the Nephrotic Syndrome

"CRAMMING FACTS"

Congenital.

Renal artery or vein thrombosis, inferior vena cava thrombosis.

Auto-immune: SLE, polyarteritis, Henoch-Schönlein purpura, Sjögren's syndrome.

Metabolic: myxoedema, diabetes mellitus (Kimmelstiel-Wilson).

Mechanical: IVC, thrombosis, CCF, constrictive pericarditis, chyluria.

Infection: syphilis, SABE, staphylococcus, septicaemia, malaria.

Neoplasm: myelomatosis, reticulum cell sarcoma, renal carcinoma.

Glomerulonephritis (80 per cent): minimal, maximal (proliferative), membranous and mixed.

Familial.

Amyloidosis.

Cytomegalic inclusion disease.

Toxins: drugs, mercurials, troxidone, penicillamine, gold.

Stings (bee: hypersensitivity), ivy, pollen and smallpox.

Features of the Nephrotic Syndrome

NINE Ps

Proteinuria, small albumin molecules most easily lost.
Plasma protein falls; fluid is lost. Result of glomerular
damage.
Plasma volume drops; aldosterone is released; salt
and water are retained.
Pitting oedema — pale, puffy face.
Pleural and
Pericardial effusions occur.
Pressure of blood rises later.
Prognosis varies with the cause and the damage
suffered.
Paucity of gamma globulin lowers patient's resistance.

Note: This list is not complete.

Differential Diagnosis of
Acute Glomerulonephritis

SIX As

Angioneurotic oedema.
Anaemias. Henoch-Schönlein purpura.
Auto-immune: polyarteritis nodosa and systemic
lupus erythematosus.
Acute pyelonephritis.
Acid-fast infection of kidneys.
Acute recurrent focal nephritis (diagnosed by renal
biopsy).

Also: Goodpasture's syndrome; infective endocarditis;
tumours of urinary tract.

Glomerulonephritis

"GLOMERULONEPHRITIS"

Glomerular lesion essentially.
Loss of appetite.
Ophthalmic signs, papilloedema, haemorrhages, etc.
Massive proteinuria in subacute phase.
Emesis.
Respiratory effects: breathlessness.
Urine: smoky, casts, low output, blood urea up.
Lungs: basal crepitus.
Oedema (ankle).
Nausea and vomiting.
Epistaxis.
Pale, puffy face.
Headache and hypertensive encephalopathy.
Renal angle tenderness.
Intravascular thrombosis may occur.
Temperature elevated.
Immune disease.
Serum complement diminished.

Features of Hypernephroma

"HYPERNEPHROMAS"

Hypertension.
Peripheral neuropathy.
Elevated temperature.
Raised serum calcium.
Nausea and vomiting.
Erythema.
Polycythaemia.
Heart failure due to a-v fistulae.
Renal angle pain.*
Obstruction of inferior vena cava.
Mass.*
Albumin cells and blood in the urine,* amyloid
    changes.
Sedimentation raised.*

Note: Most of these are rare features.

May start like "stab in loin" — probably a haemorrhage
into the tumour (Sir Stanford Cade).

Causes of Acute Renal Failure

"ACUTE RENAL FAIL"

Acute-on-chronic renal failure.
Cortical necrosis and (hyper)calcaemia.
Uraemia plus infection.
Tubular necrosis, toxins, drugs, mismatched transfusions (crush syndrome).
Electrolyte depletions, shock.

Renal disease: acute glomerulonephritis, renohepatic syndrome.
Excessive dehydration in children.
Narrowed or blocked renal artery, or renal vein in IVC block.
Antepartum haemorrhage, toxaemia of pregnancy, abortion.
Lodgement of stone in ureter: calculus anuria.

Fat emboli.
Acute haemolysis.
Infection: acute fulminant, septicaemia, *Cl. welchii*, Weil's disease.
Loss of blood.

Intravenous Pyelogram: Signs of Renal Artery Stenosis

Start with S

Small, smooth kidney with sharper density, slow excretion, spastic calyces.
Ureteral scalloping (collaterals), and sometimes some atrophy.

Causes of Haematuria

"HAEMATURIAS"

Hypertension and heart failure.
Anaemias. Anticoagulants and other drugs.
Endocarditis, subacute bacterial; essential haematuria.
Malignancy and mechanical (hydronephrosis).
Adenomatous lesion of the prostate.
Tropical: schistosomiasis and malaria.
Urethral lesions: caruncle, acute gonorrhoea.
Renal lesions: nephritis, pyelitis, etc.
Infarcts and infections, including tuberculosis.
Accidental damage, including postoperative causes.
Stones.

Note: Classification, prerenal, renal, postrenal, may be helpful.

Causes of Sterile Pyuria

"CART"

Chronic interstitial cystitis (Hunner's ulcer).
Antibiotic treatments when partially successful.
Reiter's syndrome.
Tuberculosis.

Stones in Ureter

(INDICATIONS FOR OPERATION)

EIGHT Ss

Site: lower-third stones have managed to negotiate
   upper two-thirds and therefore may pass.
Size.
Shape.
Stagnation (hydro-ureter and nephrosis).
Sepsis: particularly with sepsis as kidney damage
   rapidly ensues.
Symptoms.
(Above) stricture.
Stationary stone.

Features of Cushing's Syndrome

"A BAD PHASE MA(O)"

Abdominal fat.

Buffalo hump.
Acne.
Diabetes, refractory.

Psychosis and polythaemia.
Hairy and hypertensive.
Amenorrhoea.
Striae on anterior abdominal wall.
Erythema of the face.

Moon-face and muscle weakness.*
Atherosclerotic changes occur early in disease.
Osteoporosis.

Acute Adrenal Insufficiency

"SHOCKED"

Sodium falls.
Hypotension.
Oliguria (dehydration and shock).
Colour, pale.
K: potassium rises.
Emesis.
Debility: muscular weakness.

Causes of Adrenocortical Insufficiency

"DAMP SITES"

Drugs: prolonged use of corticosteroids.
Amyloidosis.
Malignancy: secondaries — adrenalectomy for mammary carcinomatosis or Cushing's syndrome (too much excised by operation).
Pituitary hypofunction.

Septicaemia: meningitis causing adrenal apoplexy (Friderichsen-Waterhouse syndrome).
Idiopathic, possibly an auto-immune effect.
Tuberculosis.
Endocrine: congenital adrenal hypoplasia (incapable of producing cortisol).
Shock and syphilis (very rare).

Conn's Syndrome: Primary Aldosteronism

EIGHT Ps

Periodic attacks of muscle weakness: compare periodic familial paralysis.
Paraesthesia.
Polyuria.
Polydipsia.
Potassium loss.
Pressure of blood rises.
Plasma sodium rises.
Pyelonephritis likely to occur.

Addison's Disease

"ADDISON'S"

Abdominal pain, anaemia, anorexia, aldosterone deficiency.
Debility.
Dark skin and mucosae.
Insidious onset.
Sodium loss, sugar low (hypoglycaemia).
Oligaemia.
Nausea and vomiting unrelated to food.
Small pulse, small blood pressure, small heart.

Features of Phaeochromocytoma (1)

"PHASE"

Paroxysmal headache induced by movement or tumour compression.
Hypertension, paroxysmal.
Apprehensive feelings.
Sweating.
Eye: visual disturbances.

Features of Phaeochromocytoma (2)

"PHASIC MATTERS"

Pain in head, pallor, perspiration, palpitations.
High blood pressure, phasic or permanent. HMMA (VMA) 4-hydroxy-3-methoxy mandelic acid in excess in urine.
Aura may precede attack.
Sites of tumour vary from neck to pelvis.
Intermittent attacks.
"Café-au-lait spots" and neurofibromatosis in association.

Medullary carcinoma of thyroid may be present.
Adrenaline and noradrenaline produced by tumour.
Ten per cent are malignant, bilateral, or outside the suprarenals.
Temperature, metabolism and white-cell count may be raised.
Endocrine anomalies in association include parathyroid hyperplasia or tumour.
Rogitine for the alleviation of an attack.
Sugar may be found in urine (30 per cent).

Causes of Cystitis

"FRED CAN'T STOP PISSING"

Foreign body, fistula.
Rectal lesions, e.g. proctitis.
Enlarged prostate with residual urine.
Diverticulum of bladder and diverticulitis of colon and diabetes.

Cervicitis, cystitis cystica.
Appendicitis: appendix adherent to bladder.
Neoplasia: particularly carcinoma, arising in or implicating bladder.
Tuberculosis.

Syphilis, tabes dorsalis.
Tropical: schistosomiasis.
Operations: after any operation particularly in pelvic region.
Paraplegia, automatic or autonomous.

Prolapse and following its repair, and pregnancy.
Instrumentation, irradiation.
Stones.
Strictures with stagnant residual urine.
Incompetent refluxing ureteric orifices.
Nephric causes, e.g. pyelonephritis, pyonephrosis.
General debility, gorgeous honeymoon.

Causative Factors in Bladder Carcinoma

"SADIE"

Schistosomiasis.
Aniline dyes.
Diverticula.
Interstitial cystitis, and innocent tumours undergoing change.
Ectopia vesicae.

Symptoms of Papilloma of Bladder

THREE Ps

Profuse, periodic, painless haematuria.

Causes of Retention of Urine (1)

"SPLASH"

Strictures and stones.
Prostatic disease and postoperative.
Lower abdominal mass: ovary, baby, etc.
Autonomic nerve damage, following resection of rectum, cord lesions, paraplegia.
Sepsis. Acute gonorrhoea.
Hysteria.

Causes of Retention of Urine (2)

"PASSING DUTCH CUPS"

Prostatic enlargements, adenomatous, carcinomatous.
Anaesthesia, spinal.
Stricture.
Senile changes: atony of bladder muscle.
Injuries to urinary tract — complete rupture of urethra.
Neurogenic bladder: (3 A s) atonic, automatic, autonomous.*
Gonorroea, urethritis, prostatitis, with abscess.

Drugs.
Uterus: retroverted gravid uterus prolapse.
Tumours of bladder and urethra.
Clots of blood, e.g. papilloma.
Hysteria.

Constrictions around penis: phimosis, rubber band.
Ulcer of meatus in children, post-circumcision.
Post-operation: abdominoperineal excision of rectum, prostate falls back.
Stones.

With kind acknowledgements to *Martin G. Hoffman, F.R.C.S., M.R.C.O.G.*

CHAPTER 12

LIMBS

Causes of Avascular Necrosis

"SPASTIC"

Subcapsular fractures damaging blood supply.
Perthe's disease.
Auto-immune disease: DLE.
Sickle-cell anaemia.
Trauma.
Idiopathic.
Cortisone, caisson disease.

Dwarfism

"REAL DWARFISM"

Rickets.
Endocrine: Too little pituitary (hypopituitarism) and
thyroid; too much adrenal (congenital adrenal
hyperplasia).
Anaemia.
Liver failure.

Down's syndrome.
Without food or protein.
Achondroplasia.
Racial.
Failure of heart and lungs and kidneys.
Infection: tuberculosis.
Sexual precocity.
Malabsorption.

Causes of Non-Union of Bones

You need a "SPLINT"

Soft-tissue interposition. Synovial fluid dissolves haematoma.

Position of reduction: too much traction, immobilization, or movement.

Location: for example, lower third of tibia is slow to heal.

Infection.

Nutritional: vessels damaged or bone diseased.

Tumour: pathological fracture.

Curved Bones

"POOR FOOT"

Paget's disease. Pseudo-arthrosis of tibia and fibula.

Osteitis fibrosa cystica.

Osteomalacia.

Rickets.

Fibrous dysplasia.

Old malunited fractures.

Osteogenesis imperfecta.

Tibia sabre-shaped due to syphilis. Subperiosteal thickening produces an *apparent* curve, not a real one.

Causes of Pain in the Heel

"FIGHTS"

Fracture and FB.
Injury.
Gout and gonorrhoea, Reiter's syndrome.
Hard skin.
Tuberculosis or other infection.
Spur, sarcoma, or secondary. Osteochondritis.

Effects of Burns

"HEATS"

Hypovolaemia.
Exudation.
Anaemia.
Toxaemia.
Stress reaction, e.g. Curling's ulcer.

Mnemonics and Tactics

Causes of Scoliosis
(Useful Headings)

Postural. Student's scoliosis.

Compensatory. Short leg, hip disease, thoracic deformity.

Structural. Vertebral anomalies, neuromuscular disease: torticollis, poliomyelitis, syringomyelia, neurofibromatosis.

Spasmodic. Prolapsed disc.

Tumours of Bones

"MOROSE"

Multiple myeloma.
Osteogenic myeloma.
Reticulum-cell sarcoma.
Osteochondrosarcoma, osteoclastoma.
Secondaries: synovioma.
Ewing's sarcoma and other connective-tissue tumours, including fibrosarcoma, liposarcoma, pseudofibromyxoma.

Secondaries in Bone: Possible Primary Sites

"Luscious Olga brings tea to randy patients."

Lung.
Ovary.
Breast.
Thyroid.
Testis.
Renal.
Prostate.

Differential Diagnosis of Swollen Joint

"GRAB THAT GOAT"

Gonorrhoea: acute manifestations.
Rheumatoid.
Accident: torn cartilage.
Brodie's abscess with sympathetic effusion.

Tumour involvement: fracture into joint.
Haemophilia.
Acute osteomyelitis with effusion.
Trophic: Charcot's joint.

Gout.
Osteo-arthritis, osteochondritis, synovial chondro-matosis.
Acute suppurative arthritis.
Tuberculosis.

Swollen Joints

"PRODUCT"

Psoriasis.
Rheumatoid arthritis, Still's disease, Reiter's syndrome.
Osteo-arthritis.
Drugs.
Ulcerative colitis.
Crohn's disease.
Typhoid and dysentery.

Causes of Charcot Joints

Need a "SPLINT"

Syringomyelia.
Paraplegia.
Leprosy.
Injections of cortisone.
Neoplasm.
Tabes dorsalis.

Causes of Osteo-Arthritis of Hip

"OSTEO-ARTHRITIS"

Osteo-arthritis.
Senile osteoporosis.
Tumours.
Endocrine: parathyroid tumour.
Osteitis deformans (Paget's disease).
Anaemia. Haemophilia. Ageing.
Rickets.
Topical: Perthe's disease.
Hereditary: congenital dislocation of hip, particularly
    partial dislocation.
Retained foreign body, osteochondritis dissecans,
    rheumatoid arthritis.
Infections: tuberculosis, syphilis.
Too heavy in weight.
Injury follows it.
Slipped epiphysis; spondylitis, ankylosing with major
    involvement.

Causes of Osteoporosis

A.B.C.D.E.

Ageing and arthritis, rheumatoid.
Bed: immobility.
Congenital: osteogenesis imperfecta.
Diet: protein loss, protein-losing enteropathy, malabsorption or intake, nephrotic syndrome, vitamin C deficiency.
Endocrine: pituitary; acromegaly; thyroid; thyrotoxicosis; adrenal (or steroids); Cushing's syndrome; parathyroid; tumours; ovaries; menopause.

Causes of Back-Ache

"OSTEOPOROSIS"

Osteoporosis.
Syphilis and shingles.
Trauma and tumours, include multiple myelomata.
Endocrine: osteitis fibrosa cystica.
Osteochondritis.
Paget's disease.
Osteo-arthritis.
Referred pain: kidney, gynaecological, pregnancy and carcinoma of the pancreas.
Osteomyelitis, include tuberculosis.
Spondylitis. Spondylolisthesis.
Intervertebral disc.
Secondaries.

Causes of Sacro-Iliitis

"STAR PUB"

Still's disease.
Tuberculosis.
Ankylosing spondylitis.
Reiter's syndrome.

Psoriasis.
Ulcerative colitis.
Brucellosis, Behçet's syndrome.

CHAPTER 13

HEAD

Features of Middle Meningeal Haemorrhage

"PEBBLE AT TOP"

Pulse slows.*

Eye: pupil on the affected side constricts then dilates,* followed by opposite side.

Blood pressure rises.

Battle's sign or bruising over the mastoid may be present.

Lucid intervals* may occur; level of consciousness is charted and falls.

Emesis may occur.

(Ataxia and cranial nerve lesions imply infratentorial haemorrhage.)

Time: two hours for dural elevation; twelve hours for bleeding from dural venous sinuses.

Tenting: uncus of temporal lobe herniates downwards through the opening of the tentorium cerebelli causing mid-brain compression.

Oculomotor nerve involvement: stretched then paralysed.

Paresis and paralysis commence on opposite side* of the lesion in majority of cases. Cerebral peduncle is compressed.

Causes of Cerebral Abscesses

"LESBIAN"

Lung infections, especially bronchiectasis.
Ear infections or operations.
Sinuses infected.
Blood-borne.
Infections of scalp or skull.
Accidents: include postoperative causes.
Neoplasia breakdown.

Causes and Periods of Onset of Cerebral Damage

"EAT IT"

Embolus: seconds.
Apoplexy: minutes.
Thrombosis: hours.

Infection: days.
Tumour: months.

Causes of Unilateral Exophthalmos

"CHEMOSIS"

Circulatory: cavernous sinus thrombosis, arteriovenous fistula (pulsating exophthalmos).

Haemorrhage into the orbit.

Exophthalmic goitre.

Meningocele.

Orbital cellulitis.

Sepsis of bone: osteomyelitis.

Invasion by orbital tumours, e.g.: compact osteoma;
glioma of optic nerve; sarcomas; secondaries, e.g.
Hutchison's syndrome (adrenal neuroblastoma).

Sinus, nasal enlargement.

Local Organic Causes of Headache

"DANGEROUS HEADACHES"

Disseminated sclerosis.
Abscesses: intracranial, orbital, sinusal.
Neoplasia: primaries and secondaries. Neuralgias.
Gumma.
Encephalitis lethargica, poliomeyelitis.
Rheumatoid or osteo-arthritis of spine.
Osteitis deformans, operative lumbar puncture.
Unhappiness and other psychological causes.
   Uraemia is an important endogenous cause.
Syphilis affecting meninges, and other causes of
   meningitis.

Haemorrhage, intracranial; hydrocephalus; herpes.
Embolus and thrombus.
Aneurysm, arteriosclerosis.
Dental disease.
Arteritis.
Cysts.
Hypophyseal tumours.
Ear: infection. Eye: infections, glaucoma, tumours.
Sinusitis.

Causes of Pain in the Ear

"LATENT"

Laryngeal, ulcers, perichondritis.

Acute tonsillitis, post-tonsillectomy, peritonsillar abscess, tumour of tonsil, retropharyngeal abscess.

Teeth: unerupted, maloccluded, infected.

Ear: infection — otitis externa and interna; foreign body.

Neck: malignant glands; neuralgia, Vth, IXth and cervical nerves.

Tongue: ulceration, including malignancy.

CHAPTER 14

MOUTH AND NOSE

Causes of Nasal Bleeding

Systemic and local. One or both sides.

"TACTICS etc."

Tumours. Primary: innocent — polyps, angiomas, fibromas; malignant — tumours of nose or antrum. Secondaries.

Accident. Picking, blowing, sneezing. Blunt injury with or without fractures of nose or anterior cranial fossa. FB with ulceration. Postoperative: ulceration from indwelling nasal tubes.

Tropical. Typhoid, leprosy.

Topical. Varices of nasal septum (Little's).

Inflammation. Acute infections — coryza, glandular fever, diphtheria, influenza, whooping cough. Chronic tuberculosis.

Allergy. Hay fever.

Collagen diseases. Periarteritis nodosa, Wegener's granulomata.

Syphilis. Gummatous lesion, rhinitis (snuffles).

Anaemias. Haemophilia, purpura, scurvy, pernicious anaemia.

Heart. Cardiac congestion. Hypertension. Respiratory tract congestion.

Reticuloses, etc. Leukaemias.

Metabolic. Uraemia, hepatic necrosis, jaundice.

Mechanical. Flying, mountaineering, diving, after violent exercise.

Drugs. Anticoagulants, cytotoxics etc.

Gynaecological/Midwifery. Pregnancy.

Dentition Sequences

MILK TEETH

"Indian ink makes cloth marks"

Incisor.
Incisor.
Molar.
Canine.
Molar.

PERMANENT TEETH

"Matron is in bed; baby comes Monday morning"

Molar.
Incisor.
Incisor.
Bicuspid.
Bicuspid.
Canine.
Molar.
Molar.

Origin unknown.

Causes of Buccal Mucosal Ulcerations

"DENTAL BRUSH"

Diabetes.
Erythema multiforme.
Noma (cancrum oris).
Trauma; brushing.
Agranulocytosis, LE.
Leukaemia.

Behçet's syndrome.
Reiter's syndrome.
Ulcerative colitis.
Sepsis, thrush, Vincent's angina, secondary syphilis,
    streptococci, staphylococci, gonococci.
Hand-Schüller-Christian disease. Histoplasmosis.

Mouth Ulcers

A.T.S.

Aphthous ulcers; agranulocytosis; angina, Vincent's.
Trauma; tuberculosis; tumours.
Syphilis; skin diseases; syndrome of Behçet.

Leucoplakia

Five Causes
1. Sepsis.
2. Sharp or jagged teeth.
3. Syphilis.
4. Spirits.
5. Smoking.

Five Sites
1. Oral cavity — tongue and cheek.
2. Oesophagus.
3. Renal pelvis.
4. Bladder.
5. Vulva.

Ulcers of Tongue

Five Ulcers of the Tongue
1. Carcinoma.
2. Gumma, deep and painless.
3. Tuberculous: these are situated on the edge of the tongue and are shallow and painful.
4. Dyspeptic or traumatic. Frenula ulcer with whooping cough.
5. Post-irradiation: these are very painful.

Carcinoma of Tongue

Five Gross Appearances
1. A warty excrescence or "cauliflower".
2. Ulcer with or without a simple rolled or everted edge.
3. A submucous nodule.
4. Fissure in leukoplakia.
5. Infiltrating scirrhous: patient is unable to protrude tongue.

Five Possible Causative Factors
1. Complicating leukoplakia.
2. Betel-nut chewing (rare).
3. Jagged-ended clay pipe (rare).
4. Associated with the Plummer-Vinson syndrome.
5. Chronic vitamin deficiency with glossitis etc.

Five Symptoms
1. Foetor oris.
2. Excessive salivation that may be blood-stained.
3. Pain in mouth or referred via the lingual and auriculotemporal nerves to the ear.
4. Dysarthria. Dysphagia (posterior-third growths).
5. Ankyloglossia.

Swellings of Floor of Mouth

Five Causes
1. Ranula. Tense, veins on surface. Treat by marsupialisation.
2. Dermoid. Doughy, softer, central site.
3. Angioma. Collapsible.
4. Cyst of Wharton's duct: associated with submandibular enlargement felt bimanually. Pain referred along tongue as lingual nerve is stretched.
5. Suprahyoid thyroglossal cyst.

Innocent Tumours of Gum

Five Localized Swellings
1. Inflammation: pyogenic acute or chronic dental abscess, pyogenic granulomata, actinomycosis (rare).
2. Tumours: including the pregnancy tumours, carcinoma, adenoma, melanoma, giant-cell tumour, papilloma.
3. Fibrous: epulis.
4. Paget's disease.
5. Gumma.

Swellings of Tongue

Five Generalized Swellings
1. Mongol.
2. Cretin.
3. Lymph or haemangioma.
4. Angioneurotic oedema or insect sting.
5. Amyloid (rare).

Five Localized Swellings
1. Lingual, thyroid, or thyroglossal cyst.
2. Dermoid.
3. Gumma.
4. Mucosa tumours: papilloma, adenoma, or carcinoma.
5. Connective tissue tumours: fibroma, lipoma, rhabdomyoma.

   Also mucous cyst and actinomycosis.

CHAPTER 15

NECK AND SALIVARY GLANDS

Causes of Parotitis

SEVEN Ds

Debilitating illnesses, e.g. uraemia. Tuberculosis, secondaries.
Dental sepsis.
Dirty mouth.
Dehydration.
Drainage by nasogastric or oral tube.
Drugs: iodides.
Diabetes.

Tumours of the Parotid

Mixed parotid tumours of varying grades of malignancy plus the following:

"A CAUSE"

Adenolymphoma.

Cylindroma: originates in duct and infiltrates along tissue planes.
Adenocarcinoma.
Undifferentiated tumour.
Secondaries.
Epidermoid.

Note: This list is not complete.

Features of Carotid Body Tumours

"CAROTID BOD"

Chemoreceptor tissue may be compressible.
Angiomatous: angiography may be useful.
Reddish-brown in colour.
Operative mortality is high (30 per cent).
Third-arch derivative, may be tender, temperature of overlying skin raised.
Ischaemia of brain with ligation of carotids is major problem: hypothermia helps.
Disseminates in 20 per cent.

Bruit or thrill may be present.
Operative removal is mandatory.
Diagnose by lateral but not vertical movement.

Lymph Nodes

If a lymph node is found, look for:

"PALS"

Primary site.
All other glands.
Liver.
Spleen.

For quick diagnosis for short cases in clinical examination.

Causes of Enlarged Glands in the Neck

"STRANGULATED"

Syphilis (rare).
Tumour secondaries.
Reticuloses.
Acute and chronic bacterial infections, e.g. tuberculosis.
Nasopharyngeal infections.
Glandular fever and other viral diseases, e.g. measles.
Uveoparotitis, undulant fever.
Leukaemias.
Amyloid disease.
Tropical diseases: trypanosomiasis and toxoplasmosis.
Ear infections.
Dental infections.

Glands above Left Clavicle

Differential Diagnosis of Malignancy
1. Face and neck: from primary oro-, naso-, or hypopharanx, larynx, thyroid, parotid, skin lesions including arm.
2. Chest level: lung and breast.
3. Abdomen: stomach, colon, rectum.
4. Entire urogenital tract: from above downwards, adrenal, kidney, bladder, prostate, testicle, ovary and uterus.

Cysts of the Neck

Five Midline Cysts
1. Thyroglossal cyst — moves with tongue protrusion.
2. Cyst of thyroid isthmus.
3. Dermoid cyst.
4. Abscess of submental lymph gland.
5. Hyoid bursa.

Five Lateral Cysts
1. Branchial cyst.
2. Cyst of thyroid lobe.
3. Tuberculous abscess.
4. Pyogenic abscess.
5. Cystic hygroma.

Indications for Tracheostomy

"TRACHEAS"

Tracheolaryngeal invasions with disease or tracheal collapse.

Respiratory mechanism depressed, e.g. tetanus, bulbar palsy, poliomyelitis.

Aspiration of the chest, if required, is facilitated by this means.

Cord injuries. Combined with other operations, e.g. laryngectomy.

Head injuries with coma.

Emergency procedure as in acute oedema, FB lodgement, diphtheria.

Accident to chest with flail segments.

Space. Dead space is reduced if necessary. 30 per cent reduction.

Complications of Tracheostomies

"TRACHEOSTOMIES"

Tracheal ulceration.
Retained secretions.
Atelectasis.
Consolidation of lung.
Haemorrhage.
Emphysema.
Obstruction due to mucous plug.
Sepsis.
Tracheal stenosis and fistula.
Over-ventilation.
Mental distress.
Innominate vessels damage.
Encrustation.
Slips out.

Horner's Syndrome

FIVE Ss

Small pupil: miosis.
Sunken eye: enophthalmos.
Slight ptosis.
Sweating absent.
Spinociliary reflex absent.

CHAPTER 16

THYROID AND PARATHYROID

"CRETINISM"

Croaky voice and cold.
Respiratory acidosis.
Effusion: pericardium.
T-wave flattening or inversion.
Instability: clumsy.
Nervous: psychosis, clumsiness, coma.
Inactive bowel: constipated.
Skin changes: thickening.
Metabolic rate reduced, cholesterol rises.

Hypothyroidism (2)

Cs

Cold, constipated, clumsy, cretinous clot with cramps, coarse skin, croaky voice, cardiac complications, high cholesterol levels, going on to coma; carpal tunnel compression syndrome may be present; cardiac complications may occur after commencement of treatment.

Cretin

Ps

A pot-bellied, pale, puffy-faced child with protruding umbilicus and poked-out tongue.

Thyrotoxicosis

"EXOPHTHALMOS"

Exophthalmos. Eyelids may be pigmented.
Ophthalmoplegia.
Palpitations. Auricular fibrillation and heart failure may
occur. Pretibial myxodaema (rare).
Hurry (intestinal), diarrhoea may be present. Hyper-
calcaemia.
Tremor, tachycardia, thrill over thyroid.
Hot hands and hungry.
Anxiety, agitation, mania. Acropachy: clubbing (rare).
Lid lag, loss of weight. LATS may be involved.
Myopathy, proximal. Menorrhagia or amenorrhoea.
Osteoporosis may occur, occasionally with vertebral
collapse.
Sweating. Splenomegaly.

Indications for Operating on Solitary Lump of Thyroid

SIX Ms

Mechanical.
Metabolic change.
Malignant change.
Mutation: any change (larger, harder), haemorrhages etc.
Marred beauty or "marriage", suggesting unsightly lump.
Mediastinal site.

Complications of Thyroidectomies

"THYROIDECTOMIES"

Thyrotoxicosis, relapse.

Haemorrhage. Suffocation may occur if it accumulates below the deep fascia.

Y

Recurrent laryngeal nerve: partial or complete injury to one or both sides.

Oesophageal damage.

Infection: from above downwards, pharyngitis, tracheitis, laryngitis, bronchitis, mediastinitis, bronchopneumonia, and wound infection.

Damage to the parathyroid glands.

Exophthalmos which may progress. Embolus, air.

Cricothyroid muscle damage.

Thyroid crisis.

Obstruction of the trachea due to its collapse.

Myxoedema.

Intrathoracic complications: pneumothorax, release of embolus from auricular appendage in patients with auricular fibrillation.

External laryngeal nerve injury.

Sympathetic nerve injury, Horner's syndrome.

Mnemonics and Tactics

Medullary Carcinoma of the Thyroid

"DAMP SCAMPI"

Diarrhoea. Note: serotonin may be produced, see
  below.
Amyloid is contained in the tumour.
Musculoskeletal effects.
Phaeochromocytoma in association.

Serotonin produced.
Cells. Calcitonin produced. Cushingoid effects.
  Calcification may be seen.
Autonomic effects.
Multiple mucosal neuromata.
Parathormone manifestations, or parathyroid adeno-
  mata present.
Inherited.

Parathyroid Glands

Classification: Too much hormone may be produced by a tumour or hyperplasia.
Inadequate amounts of hormone may result from damage or removal of the parathyroid glands.

Too Much Hormone: Hyperparathyroidism. Bent, bulging bones, with stones, abdominal groans, and psychological moans.

Too Little Hormone: Remember C for calcium, which is low.

THIRTEEN Cs

Cataracts.
Calcium low, PO_4 therefore high.
Convulsions and cramps, tetany.
Carpopedal spasm, Trousseau's sign.
Chvostek's sign — hyperexcitability of facial nerve.
Coarsening of bones.
Cracks in bone, osteoblastic activity and bone-formation may be reduced.
Character disorders, anxieties, depression.
Cardiac irregularities and arrest (cessation).
Cutaneous rashes, paraesthesia, alopecia, dry skin, brittle nails.
Coagulation of blood may be prolonged.
Calcification (basal ganglia).
Circumoral pallor, arteriolar spasm.

Clinical Features of Parathyroid Tumour

"PARATHORMONE"

Psychological: loss of initiative, anxiety, agitated depression, coma, convulsions and pancreatitis.*

Abdominal pain, anorexia, nausea, vomiting, constipation, peptic ulcer.

Renal stones,* infection, haematuria, renal failure, polyuria, polydipsia.

Arthropathy: chondrocalcinosis.

Teeth: loss of lamina dura. Tiredness.

Hypotonicity of muscles, myopathy.

Ocular: calcifications in cornea.

Rarefaction of bones, pain, bending,* fractures.

Metabolic changes: hypercalcaemia, hypercalciuria, hypophosphataemia, raised alkaline phosphatase.

Osteitis fibrosa cystica generalisata, cysts, pathological fractures and curved bones.

Nephrocalcinosis.

Erosion of phalanges, ECG changes (short Q-T interval).

Causes of Hypercalcaemia (1)

"CO-SPASM"

Chronic renal failure. (Parathyroid glands are second-
 arily stimulated due to the low calcium.)
Overdose or oversensitivity to vitamin D. Over-
 activity of thyroid.
Secondaries.
Parathyroid disease.
Alkali-milk syndrome.
Sarcoidosis.
Myelomatosis.

Causes of Hypercalcaemia (2)

"THE MAD PHYSICIAN"

Tertiary hyperparathyroidism.
Hyperthyroidism.
Excess intake of alkalis and milk.

Multiple myelomata.
Addison's disease.
D — hypervitaminosis D.

Paget's disease with bed rest.
Hyperparathyroidism, primary or secondary (renal
 damage).
Y — young: idiopathic hypercalcaemia.
Sarcoidosis.
Immobility.
Carcinomatosis.
Idiopathic in adult.
Acromegaly (rarely). Nodes, Hodgkin's disease.

Causes of Hypercalciuria

"DISEASE"

Diet: vitamin D excess.
Idiopathic.
Stasis: immobilization.
Endocrine (1): hyperparathyroidism.
Alkali-milk syndrome.
Sarcoidosis.
Endocrine (2): Cushing's syndrome.

Causes of Tetany

"REMAKE"

Renal tubular acidosis.
Endocrine: hypoplasia or removal of parathyroid.
Malabsorption: note lack of vitamin D.
Alkalosis: metabolic or respiratory.
Kidney failure: uraemia.
Excess phosphates by mouth in the treatment of hypercalcaemia.

CHAPTER 17

SYNDROMES

Albers-Schönberg Disease
(Osteopetrosis, Marble Bones)

Family "FACTS"

It is familial.

Fractures.*
Anaemia.*
Cranial nerves affected, e.g. optic atrophy.
Teeth growth affected.
Splenohepatic enlargement.

Behcet's Syndrome

"BEHCET'S"

Blood: hypergammaglobulinaemia.
Eyes: iritis, episcleritis, hypopyon.
Hydrarthrosis, recurrent; arthralgia.
CNS: confusional states, brain-stem lesions, cranial nerve palsies, meningo-encephalitis, "disseminated-sclerosis-like picture".
Epithelial ulcers, mouth, vagina and sometimes rectum.
Thrombophlebitis migrans.
Skin lesions: erythema nodosum, pyoderma.

Gardner's Syndrome

"CODED"

Colonic and duodenal polyps.
Osteomas of skull.
Desmoids of anterior abdominal wall.
Epidermoid cysts with or without punctum.
Dental abnormalities.

Guillain-Barré Syndrome

"GUILLAIN-BARRÉ"

Glandular fever, virus or mycoplasma may be present.
Upper respiratory tract infection may precede attack.
Inflammatory invasion of nerve roots may occur.
Leg weakness, then arms and face.
Lower motor neurone weakness, with muscle wasting.
Autonomic lesions, hypotension, retention of urine.
Implication of respiratory muscles may occur.
Nerves are demyelinated; paraesthesiae occur.

Bulbar musculature affected.
Acute or subacute polyneuropathy is a description.
Raised protein seen in CSF.
Residual muscle weakness may occur.
Electromyography shows changed pattern after three
   or four weeks.

Klinefelter's Syndrome

"PIGS' FAT"

Puberty onset.
Infertility; note interstitial cells proliferate and pro-
   duce oestrogens and testosterone.
Gynaecomastia.
Small gonads; no germinal epithelium develops.

Feminine in contour.
Abnormal sex chromosomes.
Two X chromosomes compete with one Y.

Lindau's Disease

"BEEN PLACES"

Brain involvement.
Epithelial tumours.
Epididymal cysts.
Nephric involvement, tumours or cysts.

Pancreas affected.
Liver implicated.
Angiomata.
Cysts.
Eye involvement, the von Hippel component.
Spinal cord involved.

   Lindau's disease is basically diffuse vascular mal-
formations with multi-system involvement and epithelial lesions.

Marfan's Syndrome

"MARFAN'S"

Muscle weakness. Myopia and retinal detachment.
Arachnodactyly.
Relaxations of ligaments and joints. Lens dislocations, hypermobility.
Familial: possibly autosomal dominant.
Aorta: medionecrosis, dissecting aneurysm, aortic incompetence.
Normal intelligence, cf. homocysteinuria.
Subluxation of lens, skeletal growth anomalies (high, arched palate), spinal curves etc.

Ramsay-Hunt Syndrome
(Geniculate Herpes Zoster)

"FAILED"

Facial paresis or spasm.
Auricular or anterior fauces vesicles.
Ipsilateral loss of taste, anterior two thirds of tongue.
Lurching due to dizziness.
Ear and mastoid pain.
Deafness.

Stevens-Johnson Syndrome

"DAMASCUS"

Drugs sensitivity, possible aetiology, e.g. sulphona-
mides, phenobarbitone.
Acute onset.
Males (common in young males; rare in females).
Acute fever.
Systemic upset.
Cutaneous purpura.
Ulceration of mucosae: mouth, eye, urethra, vagina,
alimentary tract with haemorrhage.
Severity great; the disease is often fatal.

Reiter's Syndrome

"PUB RAID"

Pyuria, non-specific.
Urethritis.
Balanitis, circinate.

Rashes. Examine soles of feet.
Arthritis, ankylosing spondylitis. Aortic valve lesion.
Iritis, conjunctivitis.
Diarrhoea may precede.

CHAPTER 18

BLOOD DISEASE

Causes of Leucopenia with
Relative Lymphocytosis

A.E.I.O.U.

Acid-fast infection.
Enteric fever (typhoid).
Infections from viruses.
Overwhelming infection.
Undulant fever.

Note: This list is not complete. Add drugs, congenital form, etc.

Factors Affecting Bone Marrow

"CAGE OF BAIT"

C – vitamin.
ACTH.
Growth hormone.
Erythropoietin.

Oxygen.
Folic acid.

B_{12} and B_6 vitamins.
Adrenal.
Iron, cobalt and copper.
Thyroxin.

Hereditary Spherocytosis

"BUGGARS"

Bilirubin elevated.
Urobilinogen raised in urine and faeces.
Girls and boys equal incidence.
Gall-stones, common.
Anaemia present.
Reticulocyte count raised.
Splenic enlargement.

Addison's Pernicious Anaemia

"ADDISON'S"

Anaemia.
Diarrhoea.
Dyspepsia.
Incidence of carcinoma of stomach increased.
Sore tongue.
Ophthalmic changes: optic atrophy, nystagmus.
Neurological: peripheral neuritis, subacute combined
    degeneration of cord.
Splenohepatomegaly.

Causes of Normocytic Anaemia

"HAEMORRHAGIC"

Haemorrhage. Haemolytic anaemia.
Aplastic anaemia.
Endocrine: myxoedema, Addison's, hypopituitarism.
Multiple myeloma.
Other malignant tumours.
Rheumatoid diseases and others.
Renal failure, uraemia.
Hepatic disease.
Ascorbic acid deficiency — scurvy.
Germs: infection.
Iatrogenic (drugs), poisons.
Cyesis.

Sickle-Cell Anaemia

"SICKLE ANAEMIAS"

Spleen enlarges and then diminishes in size.
Infarcts occur.
Crises occur with pains in muscles, bones, joints, leucocytosis.
Kids: swelling of fingers and toes, early deaths occur.
Leg ulcers.
Electrophoresis, homo- and heterozygous.

Anaemia.
Negroes principally.
Acholuric jaundice.
Epigastric pain.
Malaria-resistant.
Inherited anomaly.
American and African areas show major incidence.
Spiculation on skull X-ray.

Mnemonics and Tactics

Causes of Aplastic Anaemias

"MARASMIC"

Myeloma.
Acid-fast infection (TB).
Rheumatoid arthritis.
Antimetabolites.
Secondaries.
Metabolic: myxoedema, diseases of the liver and the kidney.
Irradiation. Idiopathic.
Chemical poisons: chloramphenicol.

Haemolytic Anaemia

Red blood cells are destroyed too rapidly in the blood or by the reticulo-endothelial system. Level of unconjugated bilirubin rises and gall-stones may accumulate; later, renal tubular deposits of iron may occur. Marrow activity increases, and premature release of reticulocytes may be seen.

Haemolysis due to Cell Anomalies

"SHIP"

Shape abnormalities: spheres, ellipses, ovals.
Haemoglobinopathies: thalassaemia, sickle-cell anaemia.
Intrinsic enzyme defects.
Paroxysmal nocturnal haemoglobinuria.

Haemolysis of Red Blood Cells due to External Factors

"CHAMPS"

Chemical: poisons, e.g. lead, snake venom.
Hypersplenism.
Auto-immune diseases, incompatible blood transfusion, haemolytic disease of new-born.
Micro-angiopathies: use of Teflon in heart surgery.
Physical agents: burns, "marching".
Sepsis, e.g. malaria, gas gangrene.

Causes of Secondary Symptomatic Haemolytic Anaemia

"MUTILATE CHARRED"

Malaria.
Uraemia.
Tumours, reticuloses.
Infections: *Cl. welchii.*
Leishmaniasis.
Abscesses.
Toxins: arsine.
Eclampsia and postpartum.

Cardiac surgery.
Hypersplenism.
Auto-immune disease.
Radiation effects.
Roasted (burns).
Enteric fever.
Drugs.

Purpuras

Haemorrhages of Mucosa and Skin

1. *Damage to vessel wall*

   (a) Mechanical: coughing, orthostatic, senile changes.
   (b) Skin disease.
   (c) Drugs.
   (d) Composition of connective tissue, scurvy.
   (e) Ischaemia of wall, caused by slowing of circulation due to globulin increases.
   (f) Allergic, Henoch-Schönlein purpura.

2. *Platelet deficiency*

   (a) Production down
   Aplasia (or hypoplasia), idiopathic, irradiation and drugs.
   Advanced malignancy — leukaemia and multiple myeloma.
   Anaemias, B_{12} and folate deficiencies.

   (b) Destruction and dilution
   Immune effects, idiopathic, drugs, infection, collagen disease, DLE, neonatal.
   Transfusions.
   Trauma: burns.
   Hypertension.
   Defibrination syndromes.

Factors Causing Purpura

"IDIOPATHIC"

Immunological.
Drugs.
Infections.
Overactive spleen.
Protein. Hyperglobulinaemia.
Atrophy of marrow.
Trauma and ageing.
Haematological: B_{12} and folic acid deficiencies.
Irradiation.
Cement problems: scurvy.

Causes of Vitamin B_{12} Deficiency

SIX Ps and TWO Cs

Pernicious anaemia.
Partial or total gastrectomy.
Pockets in bowel, diverticula or small bowel, stagnant
    loops.
Parasites: *diphyllobothrium latum*.
Pancreatitis.
Paucity in diet (vegan).

Crohn's disease, its complications and treatment,
    fistulae, strictures, bowel resections.
Coeliac disease with malabsorption.

Causes of Target Cells

"DRY CHITS"

DRY: dehydration.

Chronic jaundice.
Haemoglobin C disease.
Iron-deficiency anaemia.
Thalassaemia.
Splenectomy. Sickle-cell anaemia.

Types of Emboli

"FAT BAT"

Fat.
Air.
Thrombus.

Bacteria.
Amniotic fluid.
Tumour cells.

Felty's Syndrome

"PAUL'S"

Pigmentation of skin.
Anaemia: neutropenia, thrombocytopenia, haemolytic
   anaemia. Infection may follow.
Ulcers of leg.
Lymphadenopathy.
Splenomegaly.

Paterson-Brown Kelly
or Plummer-Vinson Syndrome

"SAD MAM"

Splenomegaly.
Achlorhydria.
Dysphagia.

Malignant change.
Atrophic pharyngitis.
Microcytic anaemia.

Causes and Features of Eosinophilia

"EOSINOPHILIA"

Eosinophilc granuloma, leukaemia.
Over 400 per mm³ necessary for diagnosis.
Skin disease, e.g. eczema.
Inherited eosinophilia.
Neoplasm: pleuroperitoneal, liver, bone, kidney secondaries, leukaemia.
Operations: post-splenectomy.
Parasites: hydatid, intestinal worms (Toxocara), filariasis, schistosomiasis.
Hodgkin's disease.
Infections: leprosy, gonorrhoea, tuberculosis, scarlet fever.
Lung: Loeffler's syndrome.
Intoxication: chlorpromazine, streptomycin, penicillin, arsenic, mercury.
Allergy, asthma,* hay fever, serum sickness.

Features of Multiple Myelomatosis

"MULTIPLE MYELOMAS"

Monoclonal gammopathy, IgA, -D, or -E, or Bence Jones protein (light chain).

Urine: Bence Jones proteinuria. Uraemia may follow tubular blockage.

Lymph nodes may contain the plasma cells.

Thrombocytopenia may complicate the clinical picture.

Infection liability is greater due to immunoglobin disorder.

Plasma-cell proliferation* is the cause.

Liver may harbour cells and may enlarge.

Elevated temperature and ESR.

Marrow biopsy is performed.

Young rarely affected.

Elevated calcium may cause abdominal symptoms: pain, constipation etc.

Limbs may be affected: paraplegia.

Osteolytic lesions.

Melphalan, prednisone, cyclophosphamide and deep X-ray therapy.

Anaemia and amyloidosis.

Splenic involvement.

Complications of Blood Transfusion

"INCOMPATIBLE"

Incompatibility.
NH₃ toxicity.
Coma, calcium deficiency may be due to citrate
toxicity.
Overloading.
Manifest hyper- or hypopyrexia.
Potassium toxicity.
Allergy.
Thrombophlebitis.
Infection: viral etc.
Bleeding diathesis.
Leaks in the system.
Embolism, air.

CHAPTER 19

VESSELS

Causes of Varicose Veins and Haemorrhoids

"TOP IN PATH"

VARICOSE VEINS	*PILES*
Tumours.	Tumours.
Obesity.	Obstipation: straining at stool.
Paget's disease and a-v shunts.	Proctitis.
INtra-abdominal tumours and abnormal vessels.	INtra-abdominal tumours.
Pregnancy.	Pregnancy.
Aneurysmal pressure.	Aneurysmal pressure.
Thrombosis of deep veins, including the IVC.	Thrombosis, leading to external pile.
Hereditary factors.	Hypertension portal.

Causes of Raynaud's Phenomenon

"TEN BARS"

                                    cervical ribs.
Thoracic outlet syndromes
                                    fixed plexus.
Ergot and other drugs.
Neurological: syringomyelia and paralysis.

Blood viscosity changes: dysproteinaemias – cryo-
  globulinaemia (macrocryoglobulinaemia, cold ag-
  glutinins), polycythaemia. Leukaemia.
Arterial disease: atheroma, Bürger's disease.
Reflex vasoconstriction. Raynaud's disease, vibratory
  tools.
Scleroderma. SLE.

Complications of Aneurysm

"STRIPPED"

Stripping, splitting, dissection.
Thrombosis: spontaneous cure rarely results.
Rupture.
Increasing pressure and damage to surrounding tissues. Infection may supervene.
Pain due to pressure or ischaemia.
Paraesthesiae, pressure on nerves.
Emboli, Raynaud's syndrome may follow distally.
Distal gangrene: patches of gangrene may be seen to occur on the limb.

Dissecting Aneurysm of the Aorta

"DISSECTS"

Double-barrelling of flow.
Ill with immediate collapse.
Sudden catastrophic pain that descends.*
Scoliosis may be found in association.
Elevated blood pressure precedes catastrophe.
Cause: atheroma, syphilis or direct trauma.
Test pulses for inequality and neurological changes.
Spinal artery damage may produce focal changes.

Causes of Impaired Circulation to the Limbs

"BE SEATED"

Bürger's disease.
Ergot and other drugs.

Spasm, Raynaud's.
Embolism.
Atherosclerosis: cardiogenic.
Thrombosis: oral contraceptive pill.
External agents: cold.
Diabetes: dehydration.

See Causes of Gangrene.

Clinical Features of Ischaemia of Limb

Ps

Pallor and pulseless, parasthesia and pain, paralysed
and particularly or perishingly cold.

Management of Ischaemic Limb

"CHAMPAGNES"

Collaterals improved by reflex heating, lumbar sympathectomy.

Hygiene: take care to avoid infection. Epidermophytosis extension, careful pedicure.

Anaemia corrected: dextran helps.

Metabolism: depressed to reduce blood demand. Cooling.

Pain: rest pain difficult to bear; strong analgesics may be required.

Anticoagulant.

Grafting: restoration of flow or by-pass.

Nerve damage: avoid trophic ulcers.

Exercises: Bürger's.

Smoking: stopped.

With kind acknowledgement to R. M. Kirk, M.S., F.R.C.S.

Causes of Unilateral Oedema of Leg

"SPINSTER"

Spontaneous, congenital, lymphoedema praecox.
Postoperative-block dissection, groin or axilla.
Irradiation, e.g. axillary for malignancy.
Neoplasm: obstructing veins or lymphatics.
Sepsis: varicose ulcer with chronic infection damages
  lymphatics.
Thrombosis of deep veins.*
Elephantiasis.
Reticuloses or secondaries.

Leg Ulcers

Leg may be "ULCERATED"

Ulcerative colitis.
Luetic, leprosy, leukaemia.
Circulatory: varicose veins, a-v fistulae, arterial
   ischaemia, lymphatic obstruction.
Excoriation.
Rheumatoid arthritis and irradiation.
Anaemias: acholuric jaundice, sickle-cell anaemia.
Tumours, tuberculosis, trophic.
Erythema induratum scrofulosum (Bazin's disease).
Diabetes, dermatophytes *(Actinomyces madurae)*.

Perforating Ulcers of Foot

"STANDS"

Syphilis.
Tropical: leprosy. Trauma.
Atherosclerosis.
Neuropathy: other causes.
Diabetes.
Sepsis: include tuberculosis.

Causes of Gangrene (1)

"DESPERATE"

Diabetes.
Ergot.
Syphilis.
Physical agents: blunt injury, penetrating injury, foreign bodies; burns, frostbite, irradiation; surgical operations and complications, e.g. tourniquet left on.
Embolism.
Raynaud's.
Atherosclerosis, aneurysms, arteritis.
Thrombo-angiitis obliterans.
Enteric fever, terminal stage.

Causes of Gangrene (2)

"TISSUE DEATH"

Trauma.
Infection: carbuncle.
Syphilis.
Spasm: Raynaud's disease.
Ulcers: trophic.
Ergot and other drugs, adrenaline, thiopentone.

Diabetes.
Embolism.
Atheroma, arteritis, aneurysm.
Thrombosis phlegmasia caeruleus (blue leg).
  Thrombo-angiitis obliterans.
Heat (excessive), frostbite, irradiation burns,
  chemicals.

Atherosclerosis – Aetiological Factors

"ATHEROMAS"

Ageing.
Toxic: long febrile illness in childhood?
Hypertension.
Endocrine: myxoedema, diabetes.
Racial. Familial.
Obesity and exercise.
Metabolic: hypercholesterolaemia. Muscle cells appear in intima.
Animal fats.
Sex and stress.

Causes of Arterial Emboli

"FACE"

Fibrillation.
Aneurysm or atheromatous plaque.
Coronary thrombosis.
Endocarditis.

Causes of Deep Vein Thromboses

"THROMBOSIS"

Therapeutic agents, e.g. oestrogens.
Heart disease.
Rise in platelets, e.g. following splenectomy.
Obesity.
Malignancy, e.g. carcinoma of the pancreas and lung.
Baby in uterus and other pressures, e.g. ovarian cysts, aneurysms, vessels.
Operations, e.g. gynaecological, prostate, prolonged operations, vascular operations.
Stasis: muscle inactivity, pressure on calf, slowing of stream.
Infection.
Senility.

Leriche's Syndrome

"LERICHE'S"

Lower segment of aorta becomes blocked.
Extremity pulses reduced or absent.
Rest relieves pain.
Iliac arteries become involved.
Claudication occurs (thighs or buttocks).
Hypertension present.
Excise clot or segment, or by-pass for treatment.
Sexual potency reduced: failure of erection occurs.

CHAPTER 20

THORAX

Causes of Mediastinal Shadows

"STAND TRIAL"

Scoliosis.
Thymic cyst or tumours.
Aneurysm.
Neoplasm including neurofibroma, teratomas, carcinoma.
Diaphragmatic herniae. Dermoid cyst.

Tracheobronchial cyst.
Retrosternal goitres.
Infections: pericardial effusion, paravertebral abscess.
Achalasia (oesophagus).
Lymph gland enlargement. Reticuloses, secondaries, etc.

Swellings in the Anterior Mediastinum

"ITS THATCH"

Intrathoracic goitre.
Thymic mass.
Swollen glands: lymphogenous cyst.

Tumours, malignant: teratoma.
Hydatid cyst.
Aneurysm.
Tumours, innocent: fibroma, lipoma.
Cysts: pleuropericardial.
Hernia: Morgagni's foramen.

Features of Murmurs

SIX Ss

Site: special site, where maximal.
Single or multiple.
Spread (conduction) and these sites.
Systolic and/or diastolic, and timing.
Soft or loud, harsh, rumbling (character).
Standing, sitting, lying, leaning, relation to exercise:
    where best heard.

Causes of Pericarditis

"IT RUBS"

Infarct: acute-extending, and injury. Posterior. MI
    syndrome.
Tumour: invasion of pericardium.

Rheumatic fever.
Uraemia.
Bacterial: acute pyogenic, tuberculosis, etc. Viral:
    Coxsackie, Benique.
SLE, scleroderma etc.

With kind acknowledgement to T. H. To, M.B., B.S.

Causes of Elevation of Jugular Venous Pulse

"BOATS PITCH"

Bradycardia.
Obstruction of right auricle by thrombus.
"A" waves (giant) and cannon waves.
Tricuspid stenosis and incompetence.
Superior vena cava obstruction, intrathoracic goitre, enlarging glands, carcinoma of lung, thymic tumours.

Pericardial and pleural effusions and constrictive pericarditis.
Increased blood volume.
Tumour in the right auricle.
Coughing.
Heart failure (right side). Hyperdynamic circulation.

Causes of Left Ventricular Failure

"ISCHAEMIA"

Infants: coarctation of the aorta.
Stenosis of aortic valves.
Cardiomyopathy.
Hypertension.*
Arteriovenous fistulae.
Excessive parenteral therapy overloading circulation.
Myocarditis or mitral incompetence.
Ischaemic heart disease, acute or chronic.
Aortic incompetence.

Management of Heart Failure

"STAMPEDE"

Sit patient up.
Treat cause if possible.
Airway should be checked: oxygen may be required.
Morphia or heroin.
Psychological reassurance.
ECG monitoring.
Digoxin and diuretics.
Electrolyte correction.

Pulmonary Hypertension

Raised pulmonary artery pressure may be caused by:
(a) increased resistance (vascular obstruction, constriction), or back pressure from pulmonary veins secondary to left heart failure;
(b) increased flow from left-to-right shunt.

Causes of Cor Pulmonale

Definition: right-sided heart disease occurring secondary to disease of lungs or pulmonary vessel disease.

A to F

Asthma, arterial obstruction (pulmonary), e.g. thrombo-embolism.
Bronchitis.
Consumption (tuberculosis).
Deformity and dysfunction of chest resulting in deficient ventilation. Kyphoscoliosis. Massive obesity.
Emphysema: impaired ventilation, structural change in vessels.
Fibrosis, alvolitis (SLE, rheumatoid), sarcoidosis, pneumoconiosis.

Blood Gases

What effects occur with low oxygen tension and high CO_2 in the blood?

Renal Effects. Aldosterone is secreted; water and sodium are thereby retained; the blood volume increases; the cardiac output rises. A "bounding" pulse is therefore discernible at the wrist.

Vessel Effects. The systemic arterioles dilate with the high cardiac output. The extremities therefore feel warm.

The cerebral vessels dilate; headache is experienced. Papilloedema may occur.

The pulmonary vessels in this condition may be constricted; hypoxia may aggravate it; and pulmonary hypertension may supervene.

Effects on Right Ventricle. The ventricle may hypertrophy initially to compensate, then dilate and fail; this process may be hastened by hypoxia; right-ventricle and pulmonary-artery enlargement may be seen on X-ray.

Effects on Blood. With low oxygen tension polycythaemia develops. If emphysema is present, cyanosis may be seen.

Note. Infection of lung causes mucosal oedema, oversecretion of mucus and possibly bronchial muscle spasm, and may precipitate acute features.

Causes of Diseases of the Heart Valves

"CRAMP"

Congenital.
Rheumatic lesions.
Atherosclerosis.
Myocardial infarction.
Pox.

Complications of Myocardial Infarction

"LAST PHASE"

Left or right ventricular damage and failure.
Aneurysmal development.
Septal damage may result in ventricular communi-
    cation, with right ventricular failure.
Tear or rupture of wall.

Pericardial effusion and pericarditis, with or without
    pleurisy (Dressler's).
Hypotension, cardiogenic shock.
Arrhythmias.
Stokes-Adams syndrome.
Emboli following mural thrombus.

Causes of Aortic Regurgitation

"CHARISMA"

Collagen disease.
Hypertension.
Arteriosclerosis and aneurysm.
Rheumatic fever* and Reiter's syndrome.
Infections: syphilis.*
SBE on congenital bicuspid valves and coarctations.
Marfan's syndrome.
Ankylosing spondylitis.

Causes of Atrial Fibrillation

"RITHMIC"

(*Note:* Correct spelling is "rhythmic", but "Y" is
almost impossible in mnemonics.)

Rheumatic heart disease.
Ischaemia: post-infarction.
Thyrotoxicosis and other toxic states. Pneumonia.
Hypertension.
Myocarditis.
Idiopathic "lone fibrillation".
Cardiomyopathy.

Cause of Systolic Murmur at Apex

"MACHINE"

Mitral valve incompetence.
Anaemia: pregnancy.
Coronary thrombosis: papillary muscle involvement
  with rupture of chordae tendineae.
Hypertension with LV enlargement.
Innocent.
Narrow aortic valve (stenosis).
Enlarged heart from any cause, e.g. cardiomyopathy.

Causes of Secondary Hypertension

"PRICED"

Pregnancy: toxaemia.
Renal causes, include renal artery stenosis.
Intracranial lesions.
Coarctation of the aorta.
Endocrine: adrenals (phaeochromocytoma, Cushing's
  syndrome or disease, Conn's syndrome) and thy-
  rotoxicosis.
Drugs: steroid therapy, contraceptive pill, clonidine
  withdrawal.

Causes of Cardiomyopathy

Primary

"PHASE"

Pregnancy and the puerperium.
Hypertrophic obstructive.
Alcohol.
Sepsis, viral.
Endomyocardial fibrosis, endomyocardial fibro-
elastosis.

Secondary

"MEDICINA"

Metabolic: porphyria, beriberi, carcinoid, Hurler's
syndrome, glocogen storage.
Endocrine: thyrotoxicosis, hypo-adrenalism, hypothy-
roidism.
Damage from tuberculosis or sarcoidosis.
Infestation: toxoplasmosis, Chagas' disease (try-
panosomiasis).
Collagen diseases: SLE, periarteritis, systemic sclero-
sis, rheumatoid, ankylosing spondylosis.
Infiltrations: amyloidosis, haemochromatosis, leuk-
aemia.
Neuromuscular: Friedreich's ataxia, myopathies.
Anaemia.

Bacterial Endocarditis

"BACTERIAL ENDOCARDITIS"

"BACTERIAL" concerns mainly the presentation and
aetiology.

"ENDOCARDITIS" relates to signs and treatment.

Bacteraemia. Blood culture, bacterial vegetations.
Anaemia, anorexia.
Cardiac murmurs, cardiac failure.
Temperature elevated.
Extraction of teeth or minor operations predispose.
Rheumatic heart disease predisposes.
Insidious onset.
Arthralgia.
Left heart mainly involved.

Emboli arterial: kidneys, spleen, brain retinae.
Nails: splinter haemorrhages, clubbing.
Damaged valves or patent ductus — already present.
Osler's nodes.
"Café-au-lait" appearance.
Aneurysms — mycotic.
Renal haematuria: flea-bitten kidney. Rash purpuric.
Duration of treatment, six weeks minimum.*
Insufficient antibiotics are ineffectual.*
Tachycardia.
Investigation: blood culture,* ESR, Hb, WBC,
complement, MSU.
Splenomegaly.*

Causes of Empyema

"SURGEONS"

Suppurating cysts or suppuration elsewhere.
Underlying lung disease, e.g. pneumonia.
Rib infections following injury etc.
Glands breaking down.
Esophageal (American spelling) perforation.
Osteomyelitis of the spine.
Neoplasm breaking down.
Subphrenic abscess.

Try "TACTICS".

Mnemonics and Tactics

Dyspnoea of Rapid Onset

1. *Four Pulmonary Ps*
   Pneumonia.
   Pneumothorax.
   Pulmonary spasm — asthma.
   Peanut or other foreign body in bronchus.

2. *Four cardiovascular Ps*
   Pulmonary embolus.*
   Pericardial tamponade.
   Pump failure (left): heart failure.*
   Peak seekers (high altitudes.)

3. *Psychogenic*

4. *Metabolic*
   Poisons.
   Pancreas: diabetes mellitus.
   Prerenal, renal, and postrenal uraemia.

Causes of Pleural Effusion

Transudates:

"SHOCK"

Starvation.
Heart: congestive heart failure.
Ovary: Meigs' syndrome.
Cirrhosis.
Kidney—nephrosis.

Exudates:

"PINK PARTS"

Pneumonia.
Infarct.
Neoplasm — primary and secondaries.
Kidney failure with dialysis.

Pleural mesothelioma.
Acid-fast infection (tuberculosis).
Rheumatic fever and rheumatoid arthritis, systemic
    lupus erythematosus.
Tropical: amoebiasis — liver.
Subphrenic infection, such as acute pancreatitis.

Causes of Pulmonary Fibrosis

"SCANDALS"

Sarcoidosis.
Cardiac.
Anthracosis. Auto-immune: rheumatoid arthritis.
Neoplasm.
Disseminated lupus erythematosus.
Acid-fast infection, alveolitis and allergy.
Luetic.
Sepsis, pneumonia, etc.

Non-Metastatic Effects of Carcinoma of Lung

"NON-METASTATIC"

Neuropathy.
Osteoporosis.
Nutty, dementia.

Myopathy, myasthenia, MSH.
Energy lack: similar to low K.
TSH.
ACTH, ADH (sodium falls).
Skin lesions.
Tremor cerebellar syndrome.
Arthropathy.
Thrombophlebitis.
Insulin effects.
Carcinoid, calcitonin.

Achalasia of Oesophagus

"ACHALASIA"

Auerbach ganglion cells absent.
Chest pain: carcinomatous change may occur.
Heller's oesophagomyotomy to cure.
Absent gas bubble in stomach.
Localization of obstruction by patient is inaccurate.
Auto-immune disease, scleroderma resembles it.
Swallowing difficult: regurgitation occurs.
Innervation of cardia is deficient: no relaxation occurs.
Aspiration pneumonia.

Rupture of the Oesophagus

"OESOPHAGUS"

Oesophagoscopy may cause it.

Emphysema occurs, is felt subcutaneously; empyema may follow.

Substernal or upper abdominal pain. Shock is severe.

Over-extension of the head during oesophagoscopy may predispose to injury.

Peptic ulcer of the oesophagus may perforate.

Haematemesis may follow. Hydropneumothorax.

Auto-emesis or emesis may cause it.

Gastric contents may be aspirated from the chest.

Ulceration due to swallowed FB may be followed by perforation.

Swallowing aggravates the pain.

Causes of Phrenic-Nerve Paralysis

"TANGLE"

Trauma: operative or due to phrenic crush.
Aortic aneurysm.
Neuritis: herpes.
Goitre: pressure effect.
Lesion of cord.
Extension of malignancy from thyroid, lung or glands.

CHAPTER 21

NERVE AND MUSCLE DISEASES

Causes of Dementia

"DEMENTIAS"

Deficiency disorders.
Ethanol (alcohol) and other drugs.
Myxoedema.
Encephalitis.
Neoplasm.
Trauma.
Inflammation.
Atherosclerosis.
Sugar low: hypoglycaemia. Senility. Schizophrenia.

Causes of Delirium

"DELIRIUM"

Drugs: ethanol, bromism.
Electrolyte imbalance.
Low PO_2.
Injury to brain.
Relapsing fever — malaria.
Infection: pneumonia, septicaemia.
Uraemia.
Metabolic: liver damage.

Disseminated Sclerosis (1)

"SIN"

Scanning speech.
Intention tremor.
Nystagmus.

Disseminated Sclerosis (2)

"REMISSIONS"

Reflexes increased.
Extensor plantar reflex.
Micturition changes.
Intention tremor.
Scanning speech.
Spasticity.
Impaired sensation.
Optic nerve.
Nystagmus.
Spinal fluid (paretic).

"DISSEMINATED SCLEROSIS"

Diplopia.
Intention tremor.
Scanning speech.
Spasticity.
Extensor plantar reflex and paraplegia.
Movement of joints reduced.
Increased deep reflexes.
Nystagmus.
Ataxia.
Temporal pallor.
Epileptiform convulsions.
Dysuria.

Sensory lesion. Loss of vibration sense.
Cerebrospinal fluid: paretic curve (50 per cent).
Loss of abdominal reflexes.
Emotional lability.
Remission, rebound phenomenon.
Optic nerve atrophy.
Sense of passive movement lost.
Impotence.
Scoliosis.

Signs of Cerebellar Lesion

"PAINS"

Pendular reflexes and hypotonia.
Ataxia with characteristic gait.
Intention tremor.
Nystagmus.
Scanning speech.

Causes of Syncope

"EACH PHASE OF MASOCHISM"

Emotional.
Anaemia.
Carbon monoxide poisoning. Coughing.
Hypoglycaemia.

Postural.
Hypercapnia.
Anoxia.
Stenosis of aortic valves.
Embolus.

Oxygen deficiency, high altitudes.
Fever toxaemia.

Micturition syncope.
Autonomic neuropathy as in diabetes.
Stokes-Adams attacks.
Obstruction by strangulation of bowel.
Congenital cyanotic heart disease.
Hysterical.
Ischaemia, cerebral.
Subclavian steal syndrome.
Myxoma of atrium, ball-valve thrombus.

Causes of Coma (1)

"CATS HATE DEAD MICE"

Cerebral thrombosis.
Alcohol.
Trauma.
Stokes-Adams attacks.

Hypoglycaemia. Hypothermia.
Aneurysm, ruptured.
Tumour.
Epilepsy.

Diabetes.
Electric shock.
Apoplexy.
Drugs.

Myxoedema.
Infections: systemic or intracranial.
Coronary thrombosis.
Encephalitis.

Causes of Coma (2)

"MAINTAINED"

Metabolic: uraemia, liver, cholaemia. Myocardial failure.
Alcohol.
Injury; includes electric shock.
Nervous: epilepsy, hysteria.
Thrombo-embolism.
Aneurysm, ruptured.
Infection: intracranial, abscess, meningo-encephalitis, septicaemia.
Neoplasia, primary or secondary.
Endocrine: thyroid — myxoedema, hypothermia; pancreas — hyper- or hypoglycaemia; adrenal — Addison's disease, adrenal apoplexy (Friderichsen-Waterhouse syndrome).
Drugs: overdose or toxic effects.

Causes of Coma (3)

A.E.I.O.U.

Alcohol, accidents, aneurysmal rupture.
Epilepsy, embolism, endocrine causes.
Infection: intracranial or septicaemia.
Overdose: opium and other drugs.
Uraemia.

Note: Tumour etc. are missing.

Nerve and Muscle Diseases

Causes of Paraplegia

"SIT FLABBERGASTED"

Syringomyelia.
Infections, e.g. tuberculosis, poliomyelitis.
Tropical: Jamaican paraplegia.

Friedreich's ataxia.
Luetic.
Accident, and those acquired before or during birth.
Blood: haematoma, spinal artery thrombosis.
Bony abnormalities:* osteomalacia, collapse of vertebra.
Escape of disc.
Reticuloses: Hodgkin's disease.
Guillain-Barré.*
Arachnoiditis.
Subacute combined degeneration of the cord.*
Tumours within or without the cord.*
Extradural abscess or cyst.
Disseminated sclerosis.*

Causes of Epilepsy

"TACTICS"

Tumours. Primary or secondary.

Accident. Birth injury; blunt or penetrating injury; FB; scarring following subdural haematoma; irradiation; postoperative scarring.

Congenital. Cerebral malformation.

Tropical. Hydatid cysts, cysticercosis.

Inflammations. Encephalitis, meningitis, abscess, tuberculosis, malaria, toxoplasmosis.

Syphilis. GPI, gumma.

Arteries. CVA, hypertension, hypertensive encephalopathy.

Nervous diseases.

Metabolic. Uraemia, hepatic coma, hypoglycaemia, hypocalcaemia.

Drugs and poisons. Lead, withdrawal of alcohol or barbituates, tricyclics.

Degenerative. Presenile dementia.

Causes of Peripheral Neuritis

"DAMNED BALANITIS"

Deficiency status: vitamins B_1 and B_{12} (beriberi, pellagra).

Allergy, serum sickness, post-vaccination and immunization.

Metabolic: diabetes, porphyria, amyloidosis.

Neoplasm: care of bronchus, myelomatosis, Hodgkin's disease.

Endocrine: myxoedema.

Drugs: Isoniazid, nitrofurantoin, chloroquine.

Blood vessels: polyarteritis nodosa.

Anaemia: pernicious anaemia, sickle-cell anaemia.

Landry's paralysis, Guillain-Barré syndrome.

Alcohol.

Nerve damage: carpal tunnel compression, Saturday night palsy.

Infection: diphtheria, leprosy, tetanus.

Thallium, lead, arsenic, mercury (Pink's disease).

Idiopathic: progressive hypertrophic polyneuritis.

Sarcoidosis, sprue, systemic lupus erythematosus.

Causes of the Carpal-Tunnel Syndrome

"GATES"

Gynaecological causes: pregnancy, contraceptive pill, premenstrual.

Arthritis.

Trauma: bruising and some repeated movements or exercise.

Endocrine: myxoedema, acromegaly, mucopolysaccharidosis (amyloid).

Scaphoid fractures.

Parkinsonism

"PARKINSON'S"

Pill-rolling. Tremor.

Ataxia.

Rigidity.

Kyphoscoliosis.

Instability, emotional and physical.

Neck muscles show rigidity and spasms early in disease.

Slow movements, stopping, slurred speech and shuffling gait.

Oculogyric crises may precede (postencephalitic Parkinsonism).

Nose tapping at its root (glabellar tap), blinking persists.

Staring and salivation.

"TABES DORSALIS"

Tabetic facies with ptosis.
Arthropathies, Charcot's joints.
Back columns of spinal cord waste, hence description
   "tabes dorsalis".
Excess cells and protein in the CSF.
Sphincter disturbances and possible loss of function.

Diplopia.
Optic atrophy.
Rombergism.
Stamping gait.
Argyll Robertson pupils.
Lightning pains, loss of ankle jerks.
Impotence.
Sensation, pain loss over "gladiator" distribution.

Myasthenia Gravis

Striated muscle tires quickly and, with rest, recovers rapidly.

Myasthenia — "MASTHENIA"

Muscle weakness.

Acetylcholine mechanism at myoneural junction disordered.

Snarling due to retraction of angles of mouth with orbicularis oris weakness. Sagging of upper eyelids.

Thymectomy is helpful in some cases. Thymic tumour or abnormality (15 per cent).

Hyperparathyroidism may be associated with it.

Eye muscle affected (50 per cent); diplopia may be present.

Neostigmine and other anticholinesterase drugs are used. Quick-acting Tensilon (edrophonium) may be used as test.

Immune factors may be involved.

Articulation, chewing, dysarthria, dysphagia etc. may worsen during day and all weaknesses may improve next morning.

Dystrophia Myotonica

"MEDICAL FACIES"

Mental retardation.
Eye: cataracts.
Dysphagia. Dimpling of tongue when tapped.
Infertility.
Children: delay in walking.
Adrenal dysfunction.
Long, haggard face.

Frontal baldness.
Atrophic gonads.
Clasping-grip* maintained. Cardiomyopathy.
Infant mortality increase.
Eye: ptosis.
Sternomastoid wasting.*

CHAPTER 22

SKIN

Systemic Pruritus

"MAD PRACTICES"

Malignancy.
Auto-immune diseases?
Diabetes mellitus, diabetes insipidus.

Parathyroid: hypoparathyroidism; psychogenic.
Reticuloses: Hodgkin's disease, leukaemia.
Allergic drug reactions.
Chronic renal failure.
Thyroid over- or underactivity.
Icterus: obstructive jaundice.
Cirrhoses: primary, biliary.
Exotic diseases: filariasis, onchocerciasis.
Syphilis, GPI.

Causes of Pruritus

"PUDDLES"

Pediculosis.
Urticaria.
Dermatitis herpetiformis.
Dermatitis: contact.
Lichen planus, simplex.
Eczema.
Scabies.

Causes of "Candida Albicans"

"TECHNICAL"

"Tropical" micro-climate.
Excess sugar in urine.
Corticosteroid and cytotoxic therapy.
Hypoparathyroidism.
Neoplasm: thymoma.
Ill-fitting dentures, inherited tendency.
Cyesis and contraceptive pill.
Antibiotics, Addison's Disease, auto-immune thyroiditis, acute renal failure.
Low iron.

Ref. *Hospital*. July, 1975. Vol. No. 7, p. 450.

Causes of Epithelioma of Skin

"BUCKLE"

Bowen's Disease.
Ulcers: chronic, Marjolin's, sinus.
Carcinogens, e.g. soot, oil.
Keratosis, senile.
Lupus vulgaris.
Exposure to sunlight, irradiation.

Differential Diagnosis of Pigmentation

"CHAMPIONS"

Cirrhosis.
Haemochromatosis.
Addison's disease.
Malabsorption.
Pregnancy.
Infestation: scratching. Pediculosis.
Overseas: pellagra.
Negroid.
Sunlight, silver, arsenic, mercury and drugs.

Skin Manifestations of Malignancy

"APPEARED"

Acanthosis nigricans.
Pachydermoperiostosis.
Pruritus.
Erythema gyratum repens.
Acquired ichthyosis.
Reticulohistiocytoma.
Exfoliative erythrodermia.
Dermatomyositis.

CHAPTER 23

OBSTETRICS AND GYNAECOLOGY

Causes of Abortion

"DEFUSED"

Drugs.
Endocrine deficiency, possibly.
Fetal abnormalities.
Uterine abnormalities.
Systemic illness.
Excision of cervix.
Damage to uterine cavity.

Causes of Amenorrhoea

"SPOUSE"

Systemic disease, acute or chronic.

Pituitary: tumours, Sheehan's syndrome, Fröhlich's syndrome, juvenile dystrophia, adiposogenitalis.

Ovary: **S**tein-Leventhal syndrome; **T**urner's syndrome; **O**vary absent; **A**rrhenoblastoma; **T**uberculosis ("STOAT").

Uterus: hypoplasia.

Sex: reproduction, pre- or post-menopause, pregnancy, lactation.

Endocrine: oral contraceptives and other drugs; thyroid and adrenal insufficiency.

Obstetric Causes of Diffuse Disseminated Coagulation

A.E.I.O.U.

Ante- and postpartum haemorrhage.
Embolus amniotica.
Inverted uterus with postpartum haemorrhage.
Old, dead fetus (may be ossified).
Uterus ruptured.

Sheehan's Syndrome

"SHEEHAN'S"

Shock, haemorrhagic, precedes syndrome.
Hair loss: pubis and axillae.
Ebbing strength.
Endocrine changes: adrenal, ovary, thyroid.
Hot weather preferred to cold.
Anterior pituitary atrophies. Amenorrhoea.
No lactation.
Skin whitens: depigmentation. Sweating stops.

Endometriosis

"ENDOMETRIOSIS"

Endoscopy useful for diagnosis.
Nulliparous patients more commonly affected.
Dyspareunia, dysmenorrhoea, dysuria.
Ovaries: chocolate cysts.
Menorrhagia, myometrial hypertrophy.
Embolization.
Tender uterosacral ligaments.
Rectal involvement: bleeding.
Infertility.
Oestrogen-dependent.
Suprapubic pain.
Intestinal obstructions, adhesions.
Scarring: anterior abdominal wall.

CHAPTER 24

MISCELLANEOUS MEDICAL DISEASES, COLLAGENOSES etc

Complications of Diabetes Mellitus

"HUMANITARIANS"

Hyperglycaemic coma.
Ulceration of legs and other areas.
Myopathy (rare).
Arteriosclerosis and hypertension: gangrene of toes.
Nephrosclerosis and other renal lesions. Polyuria.
Infections.
Thinning (loss of weight).
Autonomic effects.
Retinopathy, cataracts and other eye effects.
Insulin coma.
Acid-fast bacilli (tuberculosis), involvement of lung
  due to lowered resistance.
Nerves, including cranial nerves, may be involved.
  Peripheral involvement is usually sensory or motor.
  Paraplegia may occur.
Skin manifestations: boils, carbuncles, reactions to
  injections.

Features of Rheumatoid Arthritis

"RHEUMATOID ARTHRITIS"

Respiratory: nodules, effusions and fibrosis.
Heart: nodules, effusions and fibrosis.
Entrapment neuropathy.
Ulcers, leg.
Myopathy, motor neuropathy (mononeuritis multiplex).
Anaemia, amyloidosis.
Tendons: tenosynovitis, rupture.
Ocular: episcleritis, scleritis, scleromalasia perforans.
Inflammatory vasculitis.
Distal enlargements occur as presenting signs.

Atlanto-axial subluxation.
Rheumatoid nodules.
Thinning of the bones, periarticular and generalized.
Hoarseness: crico-arytenoid involvement.
Rheumatoid factor present.
Iatrogenic: anaemia, osteoporosis, marrow depression and bleeding.
Treatment: medical, surgical, physiotherapy and occupational therapy.
Infection may precede disease: immunological factors develop.
Systemic manifestations: fever, anorexia, weight loss, sweating, sensory neuropathy. Syndromes: Caplan's, Felty's, Sjögren's.

Extra-Articular Manifestations of Rheumatoid Arthritis

"CLEAN SPUDS"

Cardiac.
Lymphadenopathy.
Eye: episcleritis.
Anaemia and amyloidosis.
Neuropathies.

Sjögren's syndrome.
Pulmonary infiltration, then fibrosis. Pleurisy.
Ulcerated legs.
Digital vasculitis.
Skin nodules.

With kind acknowledgement to Alison Early, M.R.C.P.

Mnemonics and Tactics

Causes of Erythema Nodosum

"CUT BAD SOIL"

Crohn's disease.
Ulcerative colitis.
Toxoplasmosis.

Behçet's disease.
Acid-fast infection: tuberculosis, leprosy.
Drugs: sulphonilamides.

Sarcoidosis.
Other infections: streptococci, etc.
Idiopathic.
Lymphogranuloma venereum.

Causes of Clubbing

SEVEN Cs

Cardiac: subacute bacterial endocarditis, cyanotic congenital heart disease.

Chest: cystic fibrosis, empyema, bronchiectasis, carcinoma of lung, tuberculosis (only with extensive fibrosis), fibrosing alveolitis, abscess.

Colitis: Crohn's disease, coeliac disease, cirrhosis.

Circulatory: a-v fistula in arms.

Carcinomas: stomach etc.

Congenital.

Cervical rib (unilateral).

Also: thyrotoxicosis.

Sarcoidosis

A to U

Asymptomatic onset is frequent.
Blood: normocytic rarely haemolytic, occasional eosinophilia, hypergammaglobulinaemia.
Cardiac changes: cor pulmonale, myocardial infarction (rare), conduction defects.
Dactylitis with areas of rarefaction in phalanges.
Elevated ESR.
Fever.
Glands:* lymph enlarge; salivary involvement (Mikulicz).
Hepatomegaly.
Iridocyclitis, iritis, corneal and vitreous opacities.
Joints: arthralgia or polyarthropathy.
Kveim test positive: intradermal injection of sarcoid suspension.
Lung involvement:* hilar lymphadenopathy, infiltration and fibrosis of lung.
Metabolic changes: hypercalcaemia (25 per cent); hypercalciuria; hypersensitive to vitamin D; raised alkaline phosphatase.
Neurological changes (rare): facial palsy etc.
Oropharynx inflamed.
Pathology: epitheloid granulomata without caseation.
Q
Renal involvement, secondary to metabolic changes, infiltration (rare).
Skin: various manifestations, lupus pernio, etc.
Tubercular test usually negative.
Uveoparotid syndrome may occur.

Disseminated Lupus Erythematosus

"DISSEMINATED LUPUS ERYTHEMATOSUS"

Discoid lesions of skin, butterfly distributions on the face.
Iron and other anaemias.
Skin rashes.
Splenomegaly (rare).
Erythrocyte antibodies.
Myocarditis.
IgG raised.
Nuclear anti-factor present.
Arthritis. Simulating rheumatoid.
Tachycardia with myocarditis.
Endocarditis (Libman-Sacks).
Dilatation of the heart.

Leucopenia, ladies mainly.
Uraemia.
Pulmonary infiltration, pleurisy and pericarditis.
Under 50 years of age usually.
Seizures: epilepsy (very rare).

Emaciation: loss of weight.
Rheumatoid factor in blood.
Temperature elevated.
Hargreaves LE cells present.
Effusion in pleural cavity, or pleurisy, dry.
Myopathy.
Azathioprine for treatment.
Thrombocytopenia may occur due to platelet antibodies.
Obstructions of follicular openings in skin; horny plugs form.
Steroids are mainstay of treatment.
Uveitis, iridocyclitis.
Subarachnoid haemorrhages may cause death.

Scleroderma

"SCLERODERMAS"

Stiffness and aching. Skin feels thick and inelastic.
Calcinosis, sclerodactyly and telangiectasia (a variant).
Loss of weight.
Elevated pulmonary pressure — cor pulmonale.
Raynaud's syndrome.
Oesophagus — dysphagia.
Dyspnoea (50 per cent).
ESR raised.
Recurrent ulcers: Raynaud's.
Mouth: skin contracts. Muscle weakness.
Arthritis, acrosclerosis.
Sjögren's syndrome.

CHAPTER 25

INFECTIONS

Features of Glandular Fever

"GLASS RAISED"

Glands enlarged.
Liver enlarged, LDH elevated, sensitive to alcohol.*
Alkaline phosphatase up.
Sore throat.
Splenic enlargement.

Rupture of spleen may occur.
Anaemias occur, haemolytic or thrombocytopenic.
Icterus.
Skin hypersensitivity to penicillin.
Elevated temperature, protracted.
Distaste for cigarettes.

Complication of Mumps

"MOPE"

Meningism.
Orchitis.*
Pancreatitis.*
Encephalitis.

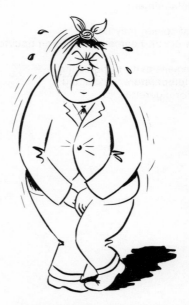

MUMPS MAKE YOU "MOPE"

Criteria for Rheumatic Fever (Duckett-Jones)

"SAFER CASES"

Sore throat, streptococcal.
Arthritis, pain, flitting, usually inappreciable physical
 signs.
Fever and sweating.
ECG changes, elevated ESR.
Rheumatic fever in history.

Carditis and tachycardia.
Antistreptolysin-O titre elevated.
Sydenham's chorea may precede or follow.
Erythema marginatum.
Subcutaneous nodules in children.

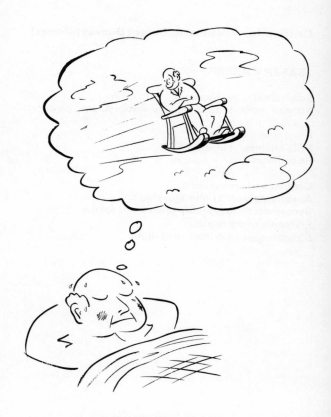

PYREXIA OF UNKNOWN ORIGIN
"THE MAGIC CHAIR"

Causes of Pyrexia of Unknown Origin

"THE MAGIC CHAIR"

Thrombosis: deep venous thrombosis, cavernous sinus (rare).

Heart: bacterial endocarditis, infarction. Haemorrhage.

Effusion: pleural, pericardial, peritoneal.

Malignancy: hypernephroma, Hodgkin's disease, reticuloses.

Anaemia: pernicious (rare), sickle-cell anaemia.

Gastro-intestinal: diverticulitis, Crohn's disease, ulcerative colitis, cholecystitis, pancreatitis.

Infection: bacterial, viral, parasitic, e.g. tuberculosis, brucellosis, typhoid, malaria.

Central nervous system damage: pontine lesion.

Cirrhosis of liver (rare).

Hypersensitivity: serum sickness, drug reactions.

Auto-immune diseases: systemic lupus erythematosus, polyarteritis nodosa.

Infection hidden: perirenal abscess, joint, bladder, dental, subphrenic.

Rheumatic disorders: rheumatic fever, rheumatoid arthritis, familial Mediterranean fever, febrile panniculitis (Weber-Christian's disease).

Try "TACTICS".

Brucellosis

"BRUCELLOSIS"

Blood cultures: IgG and IgM may be elevated; agglutination and complement fixation tests may be positive.

Reticulo-endothelial system involved.

Udders, transport route. Alternative name "undulant fever".

Contact infection: mainly an occupational disease.

Endocarditis, valve damage occurs — bacterial endocarditis (rare).

Low back pain, spondylitis may occur (rare).

Lymph nodes enlarged. Lymphocytosis with leucopenia.

Orchitis.

Splenic enlargement (in one third).

Infection by *Brucella melitensis, abortus* and *suis*.

Sweating and unexplained fever.

Rabies

"SPASTIC"

Spasms.
Pain.
Aversion to water.
Salivation and frothing at the mouth.
Temperature elevated.
Inco-ordination.
Clear mind.*

Toxoplasmosis

Nature: Protozoan, *Toxoplasma gondii.*
Commonest clinical feature: Lymphadenopathy, cf. infective mononucleosis.
Diagnosis: Complement fixation test; specific dye tests; X-ray of skull — calcifications may be seen.

Congenital:

"BIG HEADS"

Big head: hydrocephalus.
Icterus.
Granulomata, especially cerebral, cardiac either calcified or necrotic.

Hepatomegaly.
Eye: choroiditis and uveitis.
Acute fever.
Dermatological: rash.
Splenomegaly.

Acquired:

"LUNGS"

Lymphadenopathy (90 per cent).
Uveitis and choroiditis (rare).
Nervous tissue lesion: meningitis, granulomata. Necrotic nodules may be shed, causing obstruction.
Granulomata generalized: pulmonary etc.
Splenomegaly (30 per cent). Sore throat.

Effects of Secondary Syphilis

"RAW SNAIL"

Rash, maculopapular.
Alopecia.
Warts.

Snail-track ulcers.
Nodes.
Anorexia.
Iritis, iridocyclitis.
Lassitude.

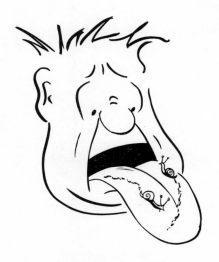

SYPHILIS. "RAW SNAIL"

Causes of Positive Wassermann Reaction

"SYPHILIS T.P." *(Treponema Pallidum)*

Syphilis.
Yaws.
Plasmodium infection (malaria).
Hansen's Disease.
Infective hepatitis.
Leptospirosis.
Infectious mononucleosis.
Systemic lupus erythematosus.

Tuberculosis.
Pregnancy.

Enteric Fever

"ENTERIC FEVERS" and ELEVEN Ps

Enlarged spleen.
Neurological symptoms, e.g., headache.
Toxic symptoms, typhoid state, semi-stupor, malaise,
  anorexia.
Enlarged glands.
Rash. Rose-coloured spots (6 days).
Infection: bone marrow, gall bladder.
Chills, cough, constipation, coma.

Fever.
Epistaxis.
Vomiting and nausea.
Excreta contain salmonella.
Râles in chest; bronchitis.
Strictures of bowel, sweating, subsultus tendinum.

Positive blood culture first few days (4).
Pulse slow.
Phlebitis.
Periostitis.
Pneumonia.
Parotitis.
Peyer's patches ulcerated.
Pyonephrosis. Premature delivery.
Perforation of bowel. Perforation of blood vessels.
  Melena and haematemesis.
Positive Widal reaction.

Gas Gangrene

"HIGH PRICE(S) TO PAY"

Hypotension.
Irregular pulse.
Gangrene develops; spreads along tissue planes.
High or low temperature.

Pulse rising is strongly indicative.
Radiological evidence of gas.
Infection with *Cl. welchii* (sugar splitter) or *Cl. sporogenes* (protein splitters).
Crepitus in tissues.
Emesis.
Swelling, smell, and sudden death*.

Toxaemia.
Oxygen (hyperbaric) is used.

Prevention by ample wound excision of dead or damaged muscle. No tension on wound.
Antisera, antibiotics and amputations (usually).
Yellow-brown exudate.

Tetanus

"STOPS TETANUS"

Swallowing difficult.
Temperature up.
Opisthotonos.
Pneumonia eventually kills.
Small stimuli provoke spasm.

Trismus and trivial injury* may precede the attack.
Excision of the wound is unnecessary; release pus if
   present.
Toxin is produced and fixes in the nervous tissues.
Active immunization and boosters advised, and anti-
   toxin employed for treatment.
Neck and back pain.
Umbilical infections: tetanus may follow. Unable to
   breathe.
Spasms and sardonic smiles.* Soil and soiled
   perineum provide organisms.

Schistosomiasis

Varieties: "A Haemorrhaging Japanese Man" *(S. haematobium, S. japonicum, S. mansoni.)*

Life Cycle.

"SCHIS"

Spined sharp eggs leave by the excreta, hatch in water, swim and enter snail.

Cercariae leave snails and with two tails enter man (host).

Habitat thereafter is hepatic; therein males and females are formed. The worms live in a variety of vessels and lay eggs. Summary is **"CHUMP"**: cystic, haemorrhoidal, uterine, mesenteric, portal vessels.

Intermediate host produces sporocyst.

Snail is intermediate host.

Clinical Manifestations of "S. Mansoni".

"CAUSE REACHED"

Colitis and cough.
Abdominal pain.
Urticaria.
Skin rashes.
Eosinophilia.

Rigors.
Elevated temperature.
Ascites.
Cirrhosis.
Headache.
Enlargements of liver and spleen.
Diarrhoea, bloody.

Infections

CHAPTER 26

METABOLIC DISORDERS

Conditions Associated with Gout

"HARD"

Hypertension.*
Atherosclerosis.*
Renal stones.*
Diabetes mellitus.

Amyloidosis

"ROUGH AMYLOIDOSIS"

Rectal or gum biopsy for diagnosis.
Onset and progress insidious.
Uraemia may follow due to renal involvement via the nephrotic syndrome (albuminuria).
Gut: malabsorption, macroglossia, dysphagia.
Heart and other muscle involvement.

Addison's disease and ascites may be causes.
Multiple myeloma may precede disease.
Yellow with jaundice.
Liver involvement.
Oedema may occur.
Iodine and sulphuric acid stains secondary amyloid blue. Employ Congo red test.
Dysarthria.
Osteomyelitis may precede disease.
Sago spleen.
Inflammation of the colon or chest (tuberculosis) are possible causes.
Suppuration may precipitate the change.

Note Primary disease in heart, alimentary tract, tongue (HAT). Secondary in spleen, adrenals, liver, kidney (SALK).

Porphyrias

Varieties: Hepatic. Erythropoietic: congenital, protoporphyria.

A to M

Abdominal pain: colicky or continuous.
Barbiturate sensitivity: the complication of epilepsy prompts possible injudicious use of barbiturates.
Constipation. Cutaneous pigmentation.
Diarrhoea.
Electrolytic disturbance associated with ADH disorder.
Fluorescence of urine in ultraviolet light.
George III's mental illness.
Haem – metabolism disorder.
Insanity: confused states occur. Incontinence or obstruction of urinary flow.
Jaundice may occur with liver damage.
Kidney excretion: urine darkens* on standing.
Light sensitivity of skin.
Motor weakness or paralysis or sensory disturbance.

Kinnier Wilson's Disease
(Hepatolenticular Degeneration)

Caused by increased absorption, or lowered excretion, of dietary copper. The increasing levels damage liver, brain and kidney.

"A CHERUB"

Autosomal recessive.

Copper and ceruloplasmin levels decreased, and excretion of copper in urine increased.

Hepatic cirrhosis proceeding to failure; liver functions are examined and biopsy is performed.

Eye: Kayser-Fleischer rings, brown rings at limbus.

Renal damage occurs.

Uric acid excretion may be raised. Low serum uric acid may be present.

Basal ganglia are involved, with rigidity, tremor, dysarthria.

Causes of Metabolic Acidosis

"ACID RISE"

Acetazolamide therapy.

Cardiac arrest, chloride absorption with ureters in large bowel.

Intestinal secretions increased, diarrhoea, pancreatic fistula.

Diabetic keto-acidosis.

Renal problems: failure, tubular acidosis.

Ineffective homeostasis — parenteral therapy.

Starvation, salicylate poisoning.

Ethyl and methyl alcohol and ethylene glycol poisoning.

CHAPTER 27

DRUGS AND POISONS

Toxic Effects of Digoxin

"SEND BEDPAN"

Slowing of pulse (undue).
Emesis.
Nausea precedes vomiting.
Diarrhoea.

Blurring and yellow vision.
Extrasystole (ventricular).
Double: coupled beats.
Pain in head.
Anorexia, atrial tachycardia.
Nervous: mental confusion.

Note Toxicity increases with low potassium (hypokalaemia) and elevated calcium.

Lead Poisoning

A to P

Anaemia.

Basophil stippling of RBCs.

Colic with no abdominal signs, and constipation.

Drop-wrist.

Encephalopathy.

Fits, especially in children.

Glucose and amino acids may be present in urine.

Headache.

Insomnia.

Jaundice appearance is simulated.

Kidney: tubular lesions.

Lead line on gums and anus.

Metallic taste in the mouth.

Neuropathy is solely motor.

Organic lead tetraethyl absorbed through the skin is most likely to produce encephalopathy.

Porphobilinogen absent from urine (compare porphyria).

Toxic Effects of Anticonvulsants

(Example: Phenytoin sodium).

"FOLATES"

Folate deficiency — megaloblastic anaemia.
Osteomalacia.
Lymph-gland enlargement.
Acne — greasy skin. Hirsutism.
Teratogenic: cleft palate, hare lip.
Enlargement of gums. Enzymic changes: liver.
Stupor. Ataxia.

Side-Effects of Steroids

"PREDNISONE"

Peptic ulcers bleed and may perforate silently.

Retention of sodium may occur causing hypertension.

Extra deposits of fat occur on face and abdomen.

Diabetes, and carbohydrate metabolism changes.

Nervous: neurosis and psychosis.

Infection-prone.

Suppression of pituitary-adrenal function may lead to
Addisonian crisis.

Osteoporosis.

Nitrogen balance: negative phase occurs, with muscle
wasting and capillary fragility.

Eye: glaucoma may be precipitated and cataracts
may form.

Effects of Hydrocortisone

"ASHAMED TO BARGAIN"

Adrenaline — potentiation of effect. In insufficiency, vascular muscle becomes unresponsive to nor-adrenaline and adrenaline, and permeability increases. These changes tend to lead to vascular collapse. The most important circulatory action is restoration of the normal sensitivity of vascular smooth muscle to noradrenaline.

Shock — inhibited. General adaptation syndrome is mediated by cortical hormones. Stress stimulates hypothalamus to effect their secretion. Hydrocortisone is effective in inhibiting anaphylactic and allergic shock states.

Haematological effect. Adrenocortical insufficiency is usually associated with eosinophilia, lymphocytosis, neutropenia and anaemia; all of which are corrected by hydrocortisone. Hydrocortisone, however, in excess (Cushing's syndrome), induces eosinopenia, lymphopenia, neutrophil leucocytosis and polycythaemia.

Anti-hypotensive. Adrenocortical insufficiency is associated with hypotension, which is corrected by hydrocortisone, partly by restoring plasma Na^+ and the circulating blood volume, and partly by overcoming myocardial weakness. In excess, hydrocortisone is hypertensive. The glucocorticoids are not such effective hypotensives as the mineralocorticoids.

Muscle weakness — occurs with excess. Muscle weakness of adrenocortical insufficiency is relieved by hydrocortisone but induced by higher concentrations by promoting loss of protein.

Electrolyte balance — effects. Hydrocortisone promotes retention of Na^+ and excretion of K^+ by the kidney and is a less potent agent in electrolyte distribution than aldosterone.

Diuretic. In adrenocortical insufficiency, there is a deficient diuretic response to water-drinking due to excessive transfer of water from the extra-cellular to intracellular fluids. Hydrocortisone counteracts this tendency.

Threshold for glucose falls. Hydrocortisone promotes gluconeogenesis, increases the deposition of glycogen in the liver, and inhibits the utilization of glucose, perhaps as a result of an anti-insulin action.

Obesity. Hydrocortisone increases the mobilization of fat and stimulates its synthesis and storage.

Bone-calcium metabolism. Hydrocortisone increases calcium metabolism; this effect together with the tendency to stimulate the breakdown of protein matrix of the bone leads to osteoporosis.

Antibody production reduced by heavy dosage.

Reduces inflammation. Hydrocortisone, in doses exceeding the physiological level, suppresses the vascular and cellular responses to injury and is beneficial in various types of inflammation. It decreases hyperaemia, reduces exudations, and diminishes the migration and infiltration of leuco-cytes at the site of injury.

Gastric juices — enriches. Hydrocortisone stimulates the secretion of several components of gastric juices. Perforation of stomach may occur during its use and may be silent.

Amino acids increase. Hydrocortisone increases the breakdown of protein; the amino acids produced are then available for gluconeogenesis.

Insulin "antagonist". Hydrocortisone excess causes hyperglycaemia, glycosuria, increased resistance to insulin and an increase in liver glycogen. The hyperglycaemia induced in man is, to some extent, compensated for by an increase in insulin secretion. Resistant diabetes occurs in Cushing's syndrome.

Nitrogen balance — negative. Hydrocortisone promotes catabolism of proteins; excess causes negative nitrogen balance accompanied by retardation of growth, wasting of muscles, thinning of hair and skin, osteoporosis and reduction in lymphoid tissue.

INDEX

Mnemonics and Tactics

Mnemonics and Tactics